Egg Pots Smoked Salmon 65

Sunshine Sauce With Broccoli Bowl And Beef 66

Bacon Avocado Salad.. 68

Ground Beef and Cabbage Stir fry 69

Snacks and Dessert Recipes 71

Keto Pound Cake.. 72

Vegan Coconut Macaroons.. 73

Keto Double Chocolate Chip Cookies 74

No Churn Strawberry Ice Cream 75

Flourless Avocado Brownies 76

Keto Chocolate Mousse (Sugar-Free) 77

Keto Pumpkin Donut 78

The Perfect Keto Lemon Curd 80

3-Weeks Weight Loss Plan: How To Lose Up To 11 Pounds In 21
Weeks? 81

DAY 1.. 82

DAY 2.. 83

DAY 3.. 85

DAY 4.. 87

DAY 5.. 88

DAY 6.. 89

DAY 7.. 90

DAY 8.. 91

DAY 9.. 92

DAY 10.. 94

KT-116-624

DAY 11...95

DAY 12...96

DAY 13...97

DAY 14...98

DAY 15...99

DAY 16...100

DAY 17...101

DAY 18...102

DAY 19...104

DAY 20...105

DAY 21...106

Disclaimer 108

THE KETO COOKBOOK

Simple and Healthy Keto Diet Recipes including
3 Weeks Weight Loss and Meal Plan

[1st Edition]

Michael Moblett

Copyright © 2019 by Michael Moblett

All rights reserved

All rights for this book here presented belong exclusively to the author. Usage or reproduction of the text
is forbidden and requires a clear consent of the author in case of expectations.

ISBN- 9781709577345

INTRODUCTION 7

Keto Diet: What Is It About?... 7

How To Use Keto Diet For Weight Loss? 8

Preparing For Keto Diet?.. 9

How To Lose 20 Pounds In 21 Days?............................... 12

Recipes.. 15

Breakfast Recipes... 17

Bulletproof Coffee Egg Latte 18

Fluffy Almond Flour Paleo Pancakes 19

Coconut Flour Crepes 20

Collagen Keto Bread 21

Keto Chocolate Cake Donuts.................................... 22

Low-Carb Keto Donuts 23

Keto Breakfast Pizza... 24

Keto Breakfast Burrito 25

Extra Crisp Cinnamon Toast Crunch Cereal 26

Oil-free Blueberry Streusel Scones 28

Keto Chocolate Muffins... 29

Buttery Coconut Flour Waffles.................................. 30

Keto Breakfast Tacos With Bacon and Guacamole......... 31

Bacon & Egg Fat Bombs 32

Bacon and Egg Breakfast Muffins 33

Lunch recipes 35

Loaded Chicken Salad 36

Zucchini Crust Grilled Cheese 37

Easy Shrimp Avocado Salad with Tomatoes and Feta.....................38

Chicken Enchilada 39

Easy Keto Lasagna Stuffed Portobellos...40

Keto Sushi...41

Low Carb Mini Mexican Meatzas 42

Spicy Kimchi Ahi Poke...43

Cinnamon Pork Chops & Mock Apples..44

Caprese Eggplant Panini with Lemon Basil Aioli 45

Slow Cooking Keto Chili...46

Keto Broccoli Soup with Turmeric and Ginger.............................47

Easy Keto Asiago Cauliflower Rice 48

Low Carb Chicken Philly Cheesesteak Bowl.................................49

Easy Keto Egg Salad 50

Dinner Recipes 51

Low-Carb Angel Hair Pasta With Lemon Chicken 52

Bok Choy Chicken Stir Fry 53

Chicken and Asparagus Lemon Stir Fry 54

Shrimp Avocado Cucumber Salad...55

Steak Fajita Roll-Ups...56

Chicken Tomato Zoodles With Spiced Cashew 57

3-Cheese Chicken and Cauliflower Lasagne 58

Garlic Chicken Creamy Tuscan..60

Baked Chicken With Tarragon Cream 61

20-minute Low Carb Turkey and Pepper.......................................62

Broccoli Rice With Chicken Coconut Curry..................................64

Keto Diet: What Is It About?

Keto diet can also be referred to as a ketogenic diet. It refers to a low-carb diet just like the Atkins diet. The main essence of a ketogenic diet is to reduce calories intake from carbohydrates and increase the intake of calories from protein and fat. It substantially reduces the intake of carbohydrates and replaces it with fat. This reduction in carbs puts the body in a metabolic state called ketosis. The body is most effective at generating energy by burning fat when it achieves ketosis.

By turning fat in the liver to ketones, the diet supplies energy to the brain. A keto diet or ketogenic diet can help to reduce insulin levels and blood sugar. In short, a keto diet is a high-fat, low carb diet. It dissipates blood sugar and insulin levels and takes the body's metabolism away from carbs to fat and ketones.

How To Use Keto Diet For Weight Loss?

1. **Include coconut oil in your diet:** coconut helps the body reach the state of ketosis since it contains MCTs. MCTs are sent directly to your liver after absorption for conversion to ketones or energy. Though it is advantageous to mix your diet with coconut oil, you should do it slowly to prevent side effects after digestion. You can start with a teaspoon daily and increase it to two to three tablespoons every day.

2. **Increase your healthy fat intake:** you should understand that a low-carb ketogenic diet doesn't just minimize carbs, but is high in fat. Consuming healthier fat can boost the body's ketone levels and help it reach ketosis. However, too much fat intake doesn't necessarily change into higher ketone levels. Fat makes up a high percentage of a ketogenic diet, supplying at least 60% calories from the fat to boost the ketone levels. Good sources of healthy fat include avocado oil, olive oil, coconut oil, butter, and tallow.

3. **Maintain adequate protein intake:** One of the mistakes that you can make with keto diet is to reduce your protein intake. Be sure you take an adequate, but not excessive protein to make your body achieve ketosis. For effective supply of amino acid to the liver, you need to consumer adequate protein ration. By doing this, the liver can then supply glucose to the organs and cells in the body that can't run on ketone. When the level of carb you consume is too low, higher protein intake allows you to sustain your muscle mass. However, you should not consume too much as it can reduce ketone production. Likewise, you muscle mass can decrease significantly when you consume too little.

4. **Test ketone levels and take the required diet:** achieving ketosis depends on the individual. The number of carbs, protein, or any other nutrient needed to achieve weight loss is not set in stones. In essence, there are different levels of nutrient intake required for each person. As a result, there is a need to test your level of ketones to see if you are achieving your goals. Ketones can be tested in the breath, blood, or urine as it will assist in determining if there is a need for an adjustment before you can achieve ketosis.

Preparing For Keto Diet?

A keto diet is pretty much different from your regular diet. Also known as Ketogenic Diet, it is a kind of diet that makes use of low carbs and high-fat diet to enable you to lose weight in a very healthy way. It involves swapping carbohydrates for foods high in fat. When this happens, the body goes into a state of Ketosis, that is the body starts to rely on the fat as it's a primary source of energy. The fat is burned into ketones that supply energy to the brain. Keto diet has proven to be very effective in weight loss because of the mechanism with which it works. Burning fat into energy requires more calories than burning carbohydrates into energy. Keto diet is also useful in treating health issues such as brain diseases, diabetes, epilepsy, cancer, and Alzheimer's disease.

A Ketogenic diet is quite similar to the Atkins diet. Some of its benefits include a reduction insulin level and blood sugar.It is also very effective in ensuring weight loss. This is made possible by the fact that a keto diet is filling and helps reduce calorie intake. The diet is composed of meals in proportions; about 70% fat, 20% - 25% proteins, and 5% carbohydrates. The goal of a keto diet is to provide another source of energy for the body, ensure weight loss and maintain the health of the individual. The body makes use of glucose as a simple source of energy and it is mainly gotten from carbohydrates. In a keto diet, the body breaks down the fat for energy in the liver, and ketones are produced as a by-product of metabolism. There are different types of Keto diet and knowledge of them is essential in preparing for the diet. Under the types of Ketogenic types, we have:

- Standard Ketogenic Diet: characterized by low carbs, moderate-protein and high-fat diet. This is the most studied and recommended.

- Cyclical Ketogenic Diet: this type of accommodates intervals of high carbs intake. Such as 5 days of a keto diet and 2 days of high carb.

- Targeted Ketogenic Diet: in this type, carbs are added to meals around workouts.

- High Protein Ketogenic Diet: this type involves more protein than the others. Although quite similar to the Standard Ketogenic diet, the protein proportion is higher.

- Moderate Ketogenic Diet: this type takes a bit of the other. Foods high in fat with net carbs (100g-150g) are consumed daily. Women with hormonal problems and some athletes have found this type quite useful.

The Standard and High Protein Ketogenic Diet are most commonly used, while the Cyclical and Targeted Ketogenic diet is used more often by athletes, trainers, and bodybuilders. The Keto diet has proved to be effective and also has some added benefits along with weight loss. They include:

1. Health Benefits: originally, the keto diet was used to cure epilepsy. This proved helpful in reducing seizures among epileptic children. Studies have shown that it can also be useful in treating a range of other health issues. Alzheimer's disease, Parkinson's disease, type 2 diabetes, Cancer, Polycystic ovary Syndrome, Brain injuries, Acne among others are some of the health challenges that are currently being treated using the keto diet. Due to the workings of the keto diet, it is effective in reducing blood pressure, blood sugar, cholesterol levels, and also heart diseases.

2. Appetite Reduction: in ensuring weight loss, the ketones produced aid in the reduction of appetite by suppressing Ghrelin and increasing Cholecystokinin (CCK). Ghrelin is the hormone that activates hunger while CCK is a hormone that makes you feel full. This would enable you to go longer without eating with your body relying on the fat for energy. This, of course, reduces the probability of overeating or taking snacks in between meals.

3. Increased Energy Levels: the energy produced from breaking down fat to ketones, are supplied to the brain. This energy is more efficient for the brain use than the one produced by glucose. This means that your body gets more energy to use as a result of the ketones. When the body is in a state of ketosis, mitochondria are created by the brain which energizes the brain cells. This increases the overall level of energy the body has.

4. Body Fat Reduction: carbohydrates are major sources of body fat which in turn leads to weight gain. Ketogenic diet ensures body fat reduction by eliminating carbohydrates and focusing on breaking down fat to produce ketones. In the absence of the glucose gotten from carbohydrates, the body slips into ketosis with reliance on the burning of fat to get energy. The body can effectively run on ketones as a source of energy.

Ketogenic diets are effective and less stressful for ensuring weight loss. The diet works with the biology of the body so it is quite advantageous to one's health. Counting calories and the likes are not necessary for a keto diet since the foods are filling and you don't need to starve yourself just to lose weight. Some of the recommended food for a Keto diet include: seafood such as fish and shellfish, cheese, low-carb vegetables, avocado, poultry (chicken and eggs), yogurt, cashew, almonds, raspberries, strawberries, blueberries, healthy oils, butter or cream, tubers, beans, grains and so on. These foods are rich and can be mixed in various ways to give delicious and appetizing meals. Ketogenic diets are somewhat therapeutic, so you should consult a doctor who will enlighten you on how best to go about it to get the desired results.

How To Lose 20 Pounds In 21 Days?

Ever considered how much easier it would be if we could lose weight as fast as we gained them? That would most definitely be awesome! As far-fetched as that might sound, it isn't completely impossible. There are ways by which you can contain and control your consumption and burn off fat to shed weight. The best part is, these methods are healthy; unlike other extreme dieting methods that don't cater to your health. It is possible to lose up to 20 pounds in the healthiest way available within 3 weeks. Of course, this would require commitment and consistency on your part. This is because losing weight can be challenging and is, unfortunately, more difficult than gaining weight for most persons. There are a few strategies that have proven to be effective and you will need to follow them religiously to see the results. Here are a few useful tips to help achieve this

1. Control your Calorie intake: as cliché as this might sound, it is the first step you'll need to take to begin the weight loss journey. Intentionally count your calorie intake and be sure to cut back on how much calories you consume. The key to this strategy of weight loss is using more calories than the ones you take in. This would mean you have to stay away from foods high in calories and fat, such as foods battered, fried, covered in chocolate or high in sugar. Stay away from junk foods. If you must purchase packaged foods, ensure you read the label thoroughly so you can maintain your calorie intake. Keeping a food journal can help monitor your calorie as it can be quite daunting doing it all from your head.

2. Take in more Proteins: these strategies aim to help weight loss so we have to ensure the body is still being nourished. Proteins are the kings of macronutrients and have been proven to aid in the reduction of belly fat and building lean mules which improve metabolism. Also, protein enriched foods are quite filing and that helps in reduction of appetite which in turn helps curb overeating. Lean protein should be consumed in every meal. Food sources of lean protein include fish, eggs, mushrooms, nuts, meats, seafood, poultry, and so on. Breakfast rich in protein sustains you longer by reducing hormones responsible for hunger and ghrelin.

3. Add Fruits and Veggies to your meals: fruits and vegetables are quite high in fiber. Fibers are very useful in weight loss because they help to slow down digestion rate such that you are satisfied without eating much. Studies have shown that an increase in fiber intake is positively associated with reduced calorie intake and weight loss. Fruits and Veggies are excellent sources of fiber. They include, apples (the peels contain the most fiber!), bananas, raspberries, oranges, mango, guava, dark-colored vegetable, broccoli, carrots, potatoes, and so on should be consumed with meals.

4. Stay off White carbs: white carbs are white carbohydrates. They are simple carbohydrates that when digested are stored as glycogen. They increase insulin and fat levels thereby causing weight gain. They are usually, processed and refined with minimal nutrient value and high calories. They tend to increase blood glucose levels and are easily digested. This, in turn, makes you feel hungry quickly and munch on snacks, which is of course processed with high calories and the cycle of weight gain commences. So you are better off without white carbs. Sources of white carbs include white rice, flour, sugar, pasta, bread, cookies, doughnuts, etc.

5. Have a food Schedule: Skipping meals do not help in weight loss as they only slow metabolism. Avoid skipping meals, especially breakfast. Breakfast should not be skipped; this is to void overeating during the day when the hunger sets in. Also, late-night eating should be avoided. Set a time after which you'd no longer eat anything. It is also important to take foods in correct proportions; 40% carbs, 40% protein, and 20% fat. Eat foods in moderation. You can do this by using a smaller plate to eat instead of larger ones and try to avoid second servings. Remember, commitment and discipline are crucial towards achieving your goal.

6. Increase your Water intake: water is calories free; so you can take as much of it and still be sure you're safe. Most importantly, water helps get rid of toxins by flushing them out thereby making it easier to lose some weight. Drinking more water is one of the easiest ways of losing weight that requires minimal effort. It also boosts metabolism which in turn increases the calories you burn after eating. Drinking water has other benefits such as keeping you hydrated, preventing constipation and maintaining internal PH. Taking 2-3 liters of water each day is very much advisable and you should take at least 2 glasses of water every morning when you wake up. Water is quite filling, so taking a lot of does help in the reduction of appetite.

7. Start Aerobic exercises: aerobic exercise is an efficient way to burn calories. Aerobic exercises are also known as cardio and they involve physical activities that help strengthen your heart and lungs. Most aerobic exercises burn between 200 – 600 calories per hour, depending on how vigorous the activities are. Aerobic exercises include running, swimming, basketball, dancing, bicycling, jumping rope, lifting a weight and so on. Try to engage in any form of aerobic exercise for at least 30 minutes every day.

8. Have a Good Night sleep: studies have shown that sleep deprivation could lead to weight gain as a result of increased hunger. After a long day's work and energy burned, the body does need rest. Having quality sleep at night is very much important to ensuring weight loss. At least 7 hours of sleep is required for the best to rest properly and function effectively the following day.

Losing 20 pounds in 3 weeks is no joke. As possible as it is, it does require a lot of hard work, self-discipline, and commitment. Losing weight and doing so healthily is very much achievable if you follow the tips mentioned above. Think of it as a form of delayed gratification that holds promising results.

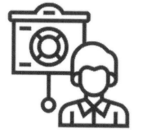

Time: 12 minutes

Amount: 1 serving

Calories: 331Kcal

Carbs: 4.5g

Protein: 24g

Fat: 25g

INGREDIENTS:

- Black coffee (8 oz/227g)
- Grass-fed butter or ghee (1 to 2 tbsp)
- Brain octane oil (1 to 2 tbsp)
- Pastured raised egg-2 eggs
- Vanilla collagen protein (1 scoop)
- Ceylon Cinnamon (1/4 teaspoon)

HOW TO COOK

1. Blend eggs, oil, butter, and mix with cinnamon
2. Add coffee then blend for 45 seconds more on high speed
3. Include collagen protein then blend for 5 more seconds at low speed
4. Add cinnamon for topping

Time: 15 minutes

Amount: 4 Servings

Calories: 341 kcal

Carbs: 8.5g

Protein: 13.24

Fat: 25.5g

INGREDIENTS:

- Blanchedalmond flour (1 ½ cup)
- ½ tablespoon Baking soda
- 1 tablespoon of Cinnamon
- 1/4 cup of pure Coconut milk
- ¼ tablespoon of Sea salt
- 3 large Pastured eggs
- (1 tablespoon) Coconut oil or Unsaltedbutter
- (1/4 tablespoon) Apple cider vinegar
- Vanilla extract (2 tsp)

HOW TO COOK

1. Preheat your griddle over medium-high heat and grease with the butter or coconut oil

2. Blend all your liquid ingredient in a blender. Place all dry ingredients on top, cover, then blend. Start at low speed then gradually increase blend speed to high. Blend for 1 minute

3. Ladle batter onto the griddle in spoonfuls until it forms a pancake of about 3" diameter or the the size of a silver dolar

4. When the batter begins to bubble, flip once

5. Repeat this until you are done with all the batter

Time: 25 minutes

Amount: 6 Crepes

Calories: 108kcal

Carbohydrates: 2.5g

Protein: 4.6g

Fat: 8.9g

INGREDIENTS

- Eggs (4 large)
- 1 tablespoonMelted virgincoconut oil
- ¼ cup Water or milk
- Melted cream (1/4 cup)
- 2 tablespoons Coconut flour
- 2 tablespoons Almond flour

HOW TO COOK

1. Mix all your ingredients in a mixing bowl. Follow this order: Pour in the eggs first, then the melted coconut oil. Add the coconut cream, almond milk, and vanilla extract before adding coconut flour then the almond meal

2. Use a whisk or an electric mixer to mix all the ingredients. Mix all until a smooth batter is formed that has no lump in it. Set aside till the coconut flour soaks for about or the batter and the liquid thickens slightly or for 10 mins.

3. Heat a mini egg plan and oil lightly. Rub the pan using an absorbent paper after oiling.

4. Pour ¼ cup at a time crepe in the batter. Tip then rotate the pan gently to let the batter spread as thinly as possible. Cook both sides for about 3 minutes on each side until crispy or brown. The crepes should unstick from the pan quite easily. Ensure that the center is set and dry before flipping or it will break.

5. To be served hot with favorite filling

Time: 1 hr 50 minutes

Amount:12 slices

Calories: 77kcal

Carbs: 1g

Protein: 7g

Fat: 5g

INGREDIENTS:

- ½ cup Collagen Protein-Unflavored, Grass-Fed
- Almond flour
- Pastured eggs (5, separated)
- Unflavored coconut oil (1 tablespoon)
- 1 tablespoon Baking powder
- Xanthan gum (1 tsp)
- Himalayan salt
- Stevia (optional)

HOW TO COOK

1. Oil the bottom of a standard size loaf dish (glass or ceramic). You can use coconut oil, butter or ghee for this or simply lay a piece of parchment paper at the bottom of the dish.

2. Set a pot aside after beating the egg whites in a large bowl till a stiff peaks starts to form.

3. Use a bowl to mix all the dry ingredients. Add a pinch of stevia (optional)

4. Whisk wet ingredients in another small bowl

5. Add to the egg whites both the wet and dry ingredients. Mix thoroughly until the batter is thick and a bit gooey

6. Prepare an oiled or lined dish and pour the batter into it. Then place the prepared dish into an oven and let it stay heated for about 40 minutes.

7. Let it cool for about 2 hours after you remove it from the oven.

8. Remove cooled bread from the baking dish using a knife.

9. Cut into 12 slices and serve

Time: 33 minutes

Amount: 8 servings

Calories: 123kcal

Carbs:4.6g

Protein: 4.3g

Fat: 9.2g

INGREDIENTS:

For donuts:

- 1/3 cup Coconut flour
- Cocoa powder (3 tbsp)
- Baking powder (1 tsp)
- 1/3 cup Swerve sweetener
- ¼ tablespoon Salt

- Eggs (4 large)
- Brewed coffee (6 tbsp) or water coffee
- ¼ cup vanilla extract Melted butter

For glaze:

- Swerve Sweetener (1/4 cup)
- 1 tablespoon Cocoapowder
- 1 tablespoon Heavy cream

- ¼ tablespoon Vanilla extract
- Water (2 tablespoons)

HOW TO COOK

For Donuts:

1. Set oven at 160 degrees Celsius or 325 degree farenheit

2. Whisk coconut flour, cocoa powder and sweetener in a medium bowl

3. Stir the vanilla extract, melted butter, and eggs. Add the cold coffee and mix it well.

4. Separate the batter into a donut pan. Place the pan in the oven and let it bake until the donuts are firm or for about 20 minutes.

5. 5.Take out the pan and let it cool for about Flip out the donuts on a wire rack to continue cooling.

For the Glaze:

1. Whisk powdered sweetener with cocoa powder in a shallow bowl. Add vanilla and heavy cream to this mixture and combine

2. Add some water until the glaze things out and attains a dippable consistency.

3. Dip the top of each donut into the glaze then leave to set for 30 minutes.

Time: 40 minutes

Amount: 6 Donuts

Calories: 257kCal

Carbs: 5g

Protein:6g

Fats: 25g

INGREDIENTS

- Blanched almond flour (1 cup)
- 2 tablespoons Gluten-freebaking powder
- 1/3 cup Erythritol
- 1/8 tablespoon Sea salt
- Cinnamon (1 tsp)
- ¼ cup Melted unsalted butter
- Almond milk (unsweetened) 1/4 cup
- Vanilla extract (1/2tsp)
- Eggs (2, Large)

For Cinnamon Coating

- ½ cup Erythritol
- 3 tablespoons Melted unsalted butter
- 1 tablespoon Cinnamon

HOW TO COOK

1. Preheat your oven to 350OF or 180OC and grease the donut pan
2. In a bowl, stir almond flour, erythritol, sea salt, baking powder and cinnamon.
3. Mix melted butter, almond milk, vanilla extract and egg in another bowl.
4. Combine the wet mixture and the dry one
5. Transfer batter into donut pan until the pan is about 3/4 of its size filled
6. 6.Bake for about 23 to 29 minutes in preheated oven until the donut turns a dark golden brown color
7. Cool donuts until they are easy to remove from pan
8. To prepare the cinnamon coating, mix cinnamon and erythritol in a bowl.
9. Transfer cooled donuts to a prepared cutting board and brush both sides with butter. Press or roll each donut into the cinnamon mixture.

Time: 25 minutes

Amount: 2 servings

Calories: 454 kcal

Carbs:26g

Protein:24g

Fat: 35g

INGREDIENTS

- ♦ 2 cups Gratedcauliflower
- ♦ ½ tablespoon Salt
- ♦ 2 tablespoons Coconut flour
- ♦ 4 eggs
- ♦ ½ tablespoon Salt
- ♦ 1 tablespoon Psyllium husk powder
- ♦ Smoked salmon, herbs, spinach, olive oil as topping and avocado

HOW TO COOK

1. Preheat oven to 350oF or 170oC. Line a sheet pan or pizza tray with some parchment paper

2. Add all the ingredients in a mixing bowl apart from the toppings. Mix until it is combined and leave it for 5 minutes.

3. Carefully power mixture onto a pan then mould into a round and even pizza crust with your hands

4. Bake in the oven for about 15 minutes and leave until it is fully cooked.

5. Take it out of the open and use it with any topping of your choice. Enjoy warm.

Time: 7 minutes

Amount: 1 Burrito

Calories: 33kcal

Carbs: 1g

Fat:30g

Protein: 11g

INGREDIENTS

- ◆ 1 tablespoon Butter
- ◆ spices or herbs of your choosing
- ◆ Add Salt and pepper
- ◆ Medium sized eggs (2)
- ◆ 2 tablespoons Cream full fat

HOW TO COOK

1. Whisk eggs, cream, herbs, and spices in a small bowl
2. In a frying pan, melt butter then add the burrito egg mixture
3. Swirl the pan to Spread the burrito evenly
4. Cover and cook for about 2 minutes
5. Lift the burrito with a spatula from frying pan with a spatul
6. Add favorite filling, roll-up and enjoy

Time: About 35 minutes

Amount: 10 servings

Calories: 172 kcal

Carbs: 4g

Protein: 4g

Fat: 16g

INGREDIENTS

- 193g Almond flour
- 2 tablespoons Ground cinnamon
- ½ tablespoon Baking soda
- ½ tablespoons Xanthan gum or 1 tablespoon flax meal

- ¼ tablespoon Kosher salt
- Grass-fed butter (80g)
- 1 egg
- Erythritol or any erythritol-based sweetener (96g)

For Cinnamon topping:

- 2 tablespoons cinnamon (ground)

- 28g Melted grass-fed butter
- 2 tablespoons Swerve or xylitol

HOW TO COOK

1. In a bowl, add cinnamon, almond flour, baking soda, salt, and xanthan and whisk till well mixed.

2. Use an electric mixer to mix the cream butter for 2-3 minutes. Add sweetener and mix till fluffy and light. Ensure all of the sweetener dissolves.

3. Let the mixture mix with the egg in a mixer until it appears lightly broken. egg

4. Turn mixer to low then add in half of the flour mixture. Mix until well combined and add the other half.

5. Warp the cereal dough with cling film. Refrigerate for one hour.

6. Preheat the oven for 350°or 180°C when you want to cook.

7. Roll out dough between two pieces of parchment sheet until it is nice and thin

8. Cut dough crosswise and lengthwise into squares then prick with a small fork

9. Transfer the cinnamon toast crunch with a parchment to a tray or baking sheet. Place the tray in a freezer for 10 minutes before baking. It can last for 3 months in this state.

10. Bake until the color turns into full golden color.
11. Brush with butter then sprinkle with some cinnamon sugar.
12. Let it cool for 10 minutes and move it to a cooling rack to cool.
13. Serve immediately or store in an airtight condition for 5 days.

Time: 40 minutes

Amount: 12 scones

Calories:122kcal

Carbs:6g

Protein:5g

Fat:10g

INGREDIENTS

For scones:
- 2 cups Almond flour
- 1 tablespoon Baking powder
- 1 tablespoon Ground stevia
- A pinch of Himalayan rock salt
- 1 cup Fresh blueberries
- 1 egg
- 2 tablespoon Almond milk

For Streusel topping:
- 1 tablespoon Egg white
- ¼ cup Silvered almonds
- ½ tablespoon Ground cinnamon
- A pinch of Stevia

HOW TO COOK

1. Set oven to 180ºC or 375º F. Use a parchment papper to line the baking sheet.
2. In a bowl, mix thoroughly the stevia, salt baking powder, and almonf flour
3. In a bowl, mix the ingredients needed for ths streusel topping.
4. Add in blueberries until the flour and the blueberries are coated.
5. In a bowl, mix egg and almond milk. Add to the flour mixture th wet mixture, continue to stir until fully mixed and the dough can be kneaded with no problems
6. Shape dough to form 12 small cones then place on prepared sheet. Each cone should be ½ inch. Press the topping on top of each scone.
7. Before the color changes into golden, bake for 21 minutes.
8. Let it cool for 10mins before serving.

Time: 40 minutes

Amount: 8 muffins

Calories: 111kcal

Carbs:4g

Protein:2.8g

Fat:10g

INGREDIENTS

- Melted cacao butter (9 tbsp)
- 2 cups chopped steam pumpkin
- ½ cups Coconut oil
- ½ cup Protein powder
- Pastured eggs-3
- Cacao powder (1 cup)
- A pinch of Salt
- Coconut flour
- 2 tablespoons Apple cider vinegar
- 1 tablespoon Baking soda
- 4 tablespoons of any sugar-free sweetener

HOW TO COOK

1. Preheat oven to 350°F or 160°C
2. Add all ingredients collagen protein powder into a blender and blend till well mixed. Ensure that the pumpkin blends well with the mixture
3. Add the protein powder then blend again at low speed until well mixed
4. Prepare a pan and a muffin tray then spoon the muffin mix into it.
5. Bake muffin for about 30 minutes. Start checking from 25 mins to prevent burning.
6. Before removing from the pan, let it cool slightly.
7. It can be served alone or with coconut cream and berries.

Time: 30 min

Amount: 5 waffles

Calories: 278kcal

Carbs: 7g

Protein: 8g

Fat: 26g

INGREDIENTS

- Coconut flour (4 tbsp)
- Granulated stevia (4 tbsp)
- 5 eggs (yolk and whites separated)
- Baking powder (1 tsp)
- Vanilla extract (2 tsp)
- Melted butter (1/2 cup)
- Full-fat milk (3 tbsp)

HOW TO COOK

1. Prepare a bowl and mix egg yolks, stevia, baking powder and coconut flour.

2. Introduce your melted butter slowly. Mix well until a smooth consistency is attained

3. Add milk and vanilla to flour and butter mixture then mix well

4. Use spoons to fold whisked egg with the flour mixture.

5. Prepare a waffle maker and pout the resulting mixture into it. Cook for few minutes until a golden brown color emerges.

Time: 15 min

Amount: 2 servings

Calories:387kcal

Carbs: 9g

Protein: 11g

Fat: 35g

INGREDIENTS

- Brain octane oil (1 tablespoon)
- 2 Pastured raised eggs
- Grass-fed ghee (1 tablespoon)
- Organic avocado (1, medium)
- Himalayan salt (1/2 tablespoon)
- Organic romaine lettuce-chopped (1/4 cup)
- Cooked pastured bacon (2 slices)
- (For garnishing) Organic micro cilantro
- Organic sweet potatoes-diced and cooked (3 tablespoons)

HOW TO COOK

1. Heat small skillet on medium heat and add 1 tablespoon of ghee
2. Into the skillet, crack one egg then pierce the yolk
3. Let it cook for 1-2 minutes until it is solid on each side.
4. Place the egg on a plate lined with parchment paper after removing it from the pan.
5. Repeat this for all the eggs
6. Mash avocado along with Brain Octane oil and Himalayan pink salt in a small bowl. Divide this mixture evenly then spread on each egg taco shell
7. Top each with the romaine lettuce
8. Place half of the diced potato on each taco. Sprinkle Himalayan salt and cilantro for garnish.
9. To form taco, fold into halves.

Time: 45 minutes

Amount: 6 servings

Calories:186kcal

Carbs: 0.2g

Protein 5g

Fats: 18.4g

INGREDIENTS

- 2 large Eggs
- Butter or ghee (1/4 cup)
- Ghee (2 oz/55g)
- 2 tablespoons Mayonnaise
- Black pepper-freshly grounds
- Salt (1/4 tablespoon)
- Bacon (4 slices, Large)

HOW TO COOK

1. 1.Set the oven to 190° C or 375 °F. Line the baking tray with baking paper to prepare it.

2. Lay bacon strips flay in the baking tray ensure that they don't overlap. Let it cook in the oven for about 15 minutes till you see a golden brown. You might need more time if the bacon slice is thick. Let it cool after you withdraw it from the oven.

3. Fill a prepared sauce pan with ¾ full water to boil the eggs. Let it boil after adding salt. Dip the egg in and out of the boiling water using a spoon one at a time. Continue this for 10 minutes until the eggs are hard.

4. Prepare a bowl of cold water and put the eggs in it after boiling. Peel when chilled.

5. But butter into smaller pieces and add peeled, quartered eggs. Smash with fork.

6. Add mayonnaise and salt and pepper to season then mix well. Add in the bacon and grease and mix. Place mixture in the refrigerator until it solidifies and can be formed into fat bombs easily.

7. Crumble bacon into smaller pieces and prepare them for breading.

8. Remove egg mixture from your refrigerator and form it into six balls. Roll each of the balls in bacon crumbs then place them in a tray that can fit into the refrigerator.

9. Refigerate for 5 days in airtight container or serve immediately.

Time: 40 minutes

Amount: 12 Muffins

Calories: 69kcal

Carbs:0.5g

Protein:5.6g

Fat:5g

INGREDIENTS

- Bacon (8 slices)
- Eggs (8, large)
- Chopped green onion (2/3 cup)

HOW TO COOK

1. Preheat oven to 350oF or 160oC. Prepare a muffin tin by coating with cooking spray

2. In pan, cook bacon over medium heat. Transfer to a plate after it has cooked to a crisp. Line the plate with paper towel before transferring.

3. Leave to cool for some minutes then chop into smaller pieces.

4. Whisk eggs in a mixing bowl, add the green onions and bacon baconand green then mix until ingredients are fully combined

5. Pour egg mixture into prepared muffin tins until each cavity is half-full

6. Bake in the oven for 25mins till the edges turn golden brown.

7. Leave to cool and serve after removing from th oven.

LUNCH RECIPES

Time: 18 minutes

Amount: 4 servings

Calories: 430kcal

Carbs:6.7g

Protein:31.7g

Fat: 29.4g

INGREDIENTS

- 300g/0.6lbs boneless Chicken breasts
- ¼ tablespoon Himalayan salt
- ¼ tablespoon Extra virgin olive oil
- ¼ tablespoon black pepper
- Mozzarella balls (100g/0.2 lbs)

- Tomato (1 Large)
- 1 Avocado
- Artichoke hears (1 har)
- Red onion (1/2)
- Basil (20 leaves)
- Baby spinach (4 cups)

For Dressing:

- 2 tablespoons Extra virgin olive oil
- 1 tablespoon Dijon mustard
- Balsamic vinegar

- Garlic (1 clove)
- Black pepper and Himalayan salt (a pinch)

HOW TO COOK

1. Peel avocado then dice. Slice the onion and dice the tomato as well.
2. Pile the basil leaves then roll up and slice
3. Prepare asparagus by cutting off the stems and slicing in half. Mince the garlic
4. Slice chicken breast lengthwise. Sprinkle little pepper and salt on each side
5. Heat olive oil 1 tablespoon in an iron skiller and fry the chicken for 3mins till the color turns golden on each side.
6. Slice the chicken after removing from the oven.
7. Mix minced garlic, balsamic vinegar, olive oil, pepper, Dijon, and salt in a small bowl.
8. To a large bowl or plate, add baby spinach. Cover with grilled chicken, mozzarella, tomatoes, artichoke, red onions, basil leaves, asparagus, and avocado. Serve with dressing.

Time: 40 minutes

Amount: 2 servings

Calories: 155kcal

Carbs: 5g

Protein: 10g

Fat: 10g

INGREDIENTS

- Shredded zucchini (4 cups)
- 1 egg
- ½ cup shredded Mozzarella cheese
- 4 tablespoons grated Parmesan cheese
- ½ tablespoon salt
- A pinch pepper (black)
- 1 tablespoon dried Oregano
- **For Grilled cheese**
- Room temperature butter
- Cheddar cheese (grated or shredded) 1/3 cup

HOW TO COOK

1. Set the oven to 220°C or 450°F. Use a parchment paper to line the baking sheet and grease it.

2. In a microwave, place zucchini using a safe-dih and let it cook on high for 6 minutes. Move to a dishcloth or tea towel then twist to get the moisture out. The zucchini should be as dry as possible otherwise you end up with a mushy dough

3. Mix zucchini with egg, Parmesan cheese, salt, oregano, mozzarella cheese, and pepper. Spread this mixture on the lined sheet then shape it into 4 square.

4. Bake in preheated oven about 20 mins.

5. Let it cool for 10mins after removing from the oven and peel it off the parchment sheet.

6. Heat pan over medium heat, butter each slice of zucchini crusty bread on one side. Place the slice in a pan with the buttered side below, sprinkle with cheese and toppings. Use the remaining bread slice with the beuuered side up as the topping.

7. Turn heat down slightly and cook for 4mins or until a golden brown color begins to form. Cook and flip gently on each side for about 2-3mins.

Time: 20 minutes

Amount:2 servings

Calories: 430kcal

Carbs: 12.5g

Protein:24g

Fat: 33g

INGREDIENTS

- Shrimp (peeled, deveined and patted dry)-8 oz/226g
- 1 large diced Avocado
- 1 tablespoon Lemon juice
- Beefsteak Tomato (1, small) diced and drained

- 2 tablespoon Salted butter
- 1 tablespoon Salt
- 1 tablespoon Olive oil
- 1/3 cup Crumbled feta cheese
- ¼ tablespoon black pepper

HOW TO COOK

1. Mix the melted butter and shrimos till they are well coated.

2. Over medium-high heat, place a pan and leave it there until it is hot. To this pan, add coated shrimps in a single layer. Sear for about a minute until it begins to turn pink around the edges. Flip, then cook for about 1mins.

3. Transfer shrimp to plate. Leave to cool as you prepare other Ingredients

4. In a large bowl, combine all the ingredients that is left and the to mix it together.

5. Add the shrimps then stir to mix

6. Add pepper and salt to season

Total time: 50mins

Amount:4-servings

Calories: 568kcal

Carbs: 6g

Protein: 38g

Fat: 40g

INGREDIENTS

- ♦ 2 tablespoons Coconut oil
- ♦ 1 lbs/0.45kg Boneless and skinless chicken thigh
- ♦ ¾ cup Red enchilada sauce
- ♦ ¼ cup water Water
- ♦ (1 can, 4 oz/500g) Diced green chilies

- ♦ **For Toppings:**
- ♦ 1 whole diced avocado
- ♦ 1 cup Shredded cheese
- ♦ 1 chopped Roma tomato
- ♦ ½ cup Sour cream
- ♦ ¼ cup Chopped pickled jalapenos

HOW TO COOK

1. Set a pot and melt the coconut oil over medium heat or in a dutch oven. Sear chickeni until it is lightly brown in oil.

2. Add water and enchilada sauce. Add green chiles and onion and reduce the heat. Cover it up and let it simmer for about 25mins until chicken is well cooked.

3. Remove chicken carefully and place on a flat surface, chop or shred chicken and transfer it back to the pot. Uncover the pot and let it simmer for 10mins.

4. Set it down from the oven and serve with jalapeno, avocado, sour cream, tomato, and chees for topping. It can be served with cauliflower rice as well.

Time: 60 minutes

Amount: 4 servings

Calories: 482kcal

Carbs: 6.5g

Protein:28g

Fat: 36g

INGREDIENTS

- Portobello mushrooms (4, large)
- Whole milk ricotta cheese
- Italian sausage (4 links)
- Sugar-free marinara sauce (1 cup)
- Mozzarella cheese (shredded)-1 cup
- Chopped parsley (optional, as garnish)

HOW TO COOK

1. Brush portobello mushrooms with a dry paper towel to remove dirt
2. Remove stems and scrape brown ribs with a spoon
3. Remove sausage from casing then press into 4 patties.
4. Press one patty into each of the mushroom caps. Ensure that it goes all the way to the edges and up its sides
5. Spoon some of the ricotta (1/4 cup) into the mushroom cap. Press to the edges. Leave a dent in the center of the cap for the sauce.
6. Spoon ¼ cup marinara sauce into each of the mushroom caps above the ricotta layer.
7. On top of the mushrooms, sprinkle ¼ cup shredded mozzarella cheese. Bake for 40mins in a preheated oven.
8. Add parsley to garnish then serve while still hot.

Time: 20 minutes

Amount:4 servings

Calories: 230kcal

Carbs: 8.6g

Protein: 4.4g

Fat: 22g

INGREDIENTS

- ◆ Nori wrapper (1)
- ◆ Chopped cauliflower (1 cup)
- ◆ Avocado (1/2 medium)
- ◆ Cream cheese (1.5 oz/42.5g)
- ◆ Coconut oil (1 tbsp)
- ◆ Soy sauce (for dipping)

HOW TO COOK

1. Before you pulse the cauliflower head in a food processor, cut it up into florets. Pulse it to the size of rice.

2. Over medium-high heat, heat the coconut oil. Add cauliflower rice to this

3. Cook for about 7mins until a slight brown color begins to form. After this, pour it in a bowl and leave it to cool.

4. Cut avocado, cream cheese, and cucumber to thin pieces. Set itt aside along with the cauliflower rice

5. on a flat surface, lay down a long later of plastic wrap then lay the nori wrapper on top.

6. Spread the cauliflower rice on the nori flower and spread it to the desired thickness. Leave some room around the wrapper edges.

7. Add the avocado on the rice starting from the edge closest to you. Then add the later of cream cheese followed by the cucumber.

8. Lift the plastic wrap gently starting from the edge closest to you. Use your hands to hold the ingredients so they don't fall. Roll the nori wrapper around the ingredients without the plastic wrap.

9. Slice sushi into 8 pieces starting from the middle

Time: 35 minutes

Amount: 4 servings

Calories: 418kcal

Carbs:7.4g

Protein:39.8g

Fat: 23.7g

INGREDIENTS

- 1 lb/0.45kg Lean ground beef
- Onion (1/2)
- 1 egg
- 1 tablespoon Salt
- 1/2 tablespoon Pepper
- 1 tablespoon garlic powder

- Riced cauliflower (1 cup)
- 1 tablespoon Cumin
- Red onion (1/2, thinly sliced)
- 1 cup shredded cheddar cheese
- ¼ cup Pepper slices

To make Cilantr1o Crema (not compulsory)

- ½ cup sour cream
- 1 tablespoon lime juice

- 1 clove garlic
- Cilantro leaves (1/3 cup)

HOW TO COOK

1. Preheat oven to 350oF or 160oC

2. Chop onions in the food processor by pulsing the onion.

3. Place onions in a large bowl, add cauliflower and pulse.

4. Add riced cauliflower to a large bowl together with the beaten egg, meat, chili powder, salt, garlic powder, and pepper. Combine then split into four portions

5. Make each piece into a thin round shell (like pizza) place these on a prepared baking sheet. Do this for all of the meat mixtures

6. Preheat the oven and bake for about 20mins. Do this till the meat is cooked.

7. 7.Set off from the oven and add onion, cheese, and pepper in sprinkles.

8. Boil for 3mins to allows the cheese to melt.

9. Until each meatza, add the vocado pieces, and serve after slicing.

10. Add the garlic and cilantro to the food processor and pulse to prepare crema. Add lime cream and lime juice then pulse till well mixed for crema. Serve as a condiment with meatza.

Time: 10 minutes

Amount: 4 portions

INGREDIENTS

- Diced Ahi tuna (sushi-grade) (1 inch)
- 1 tablespoon Soy sauce
- ½ tablespoon Sesameoil
- Mayo (1/4 cup)
- Chopped onion (green)
- Sriracha (2 tbsp)
- Ripe avocado (1, diced)
- ½ cup Kimchi
- Sesame seeds

HOW TO COOK

1. Prepare a medium mixing bowl and add diced tuna.
2. Add sesame oil, mayo sriracha and soy sauce to this bowl. Toss to mix ingredients.
3. To this bowl, add kimchi and diced avocado then gently mix
4. Serve as topping for salad greens, traditional rice or cauliflower rice. It can be chopped with sesame seeds and green onion.

Time: 45 minutes

Amount: 4 servings

Calories: 455kcal

Carbs: 4.6g

Protein: 35.4g

Fat: 30.2g

INGREDIENTS

- Ghee (2 tbsp)
- Sea salt (1/2 tsp)
- Pork chops (4, boneless)
- Cut chopped chayote into ½ inch pieces
- 1 tablespoon Cinnamon
- Any low carb sweetener of choice (2 tablespoon)
- Nutmeg (1/8 tsp)
- 1 tablespoon Apple cider vinegar

HOW TO COOK

1. Melt ghee in a skillet and add pork chop. Let it cook for 5mins.

2. Flip pork chops, add chayote then sprinkle with the sweetener, apple cider, cinnamon, and nutmeg. Let it cook for about 5mins.

3. Remove pork chops from heat, place in a meal prep container to keep it warm until you want to serve.

4. 4.Boil the mixture for some minutes. Turn heat down to low, cover then leave to simmer. Stir occasionally. Cook for about 40mins, chayote should be fork tender, similar to a baked apple in texture.

5. Serve mock apples along with the warm pork chops or store in meal prep containers.

Time: 20 minutes

Amount:2 to 4 servings

Calories: 172kcal

Carbs:12g

Protein:8g

Fats: 12g

INGREDIENTS

- Eggplants (2 small with their ends removed)
- Garlic cloves (2, peeled)
- Mayonnaise (2 tbsp)
- Shredded mozzarella (1/2 cup)
- Tomatoes (2, small)
- Spinach leaves (1 cup)
- Toasted Pine nuts (2 tbsp)

HOW TO COOK

1. Heat a countertop grill or panini press on medium heat
2. Slice eggplant into half from end to end. Slice the ggplant left into pieces 1/2 inches per piece
3. Boil garlic cloves until fragrant and soft in a skillet. Add it to mayonnaise after it cools.
4. Stir in the chopped Lemon basil
5. To assemble panini, spread aioli onto the slice of eggplant. Top with the tomato slices, spinach leaves, pine nuts, and fresh mozzarella.
6. On another slice of eggplant spread the aioli mixture then place on top. Grill until the cheese melts
7. Serve hot.

Time: 8 hrs 15 minutes

Amount: 6 servings

Calories:387kcal

Carbs: 7.2g

Protein:33g

Fat: 24g

INGREDIENTS

- ♦ ground beef (1 lb/0.45kg)
- ♦ Ground sausage (1 lb/0.45kg)
- ♦ 1 medium Chopped Green bell pepper
- ♦ Diced tomato (1 can, 14.5oz)
- ♦ Tomato paste (1 can, 6oz)
- ♦ Chilli powder (1 tbsp)
- ♦ Ground cumin (1/2 tbsp)
- ♦ Garlic cloves (3 to 4) minced
- ♦ Water (1/3 cup)

HOW TO COOK

1. Brown ground beef and sausage
2. Drain. Keep half of the fat for later
3. Place cooked sausage and ground beef in a crockpot
4. Add the fat dripping and all other ingredients then mix well.
5. Cover the crockpot and cook for about 8hrs.
6. 6.Set aside and enjoy with sour cream, chesses, and green onions as toppings.

Time: 1 hr 15 minutes

Amount:2 servings

Calories: 439kcal

Carbs: 17g

Protein: 8g

Fat: 36g

INGREDIENTS

- Onion (1)
- Garlic (3 cloves)
- 1 can unsweetened coconut milk
- 1 tablespoon salt
- 1 tablespoon Turmeric powder
- Fresh ginger (2 tablespoon)
- Chopped Broccoli (2 heads, small)
- Water (1 cup)

HOW TO COOK

1. Pour half of the coconut milk into a pan over low heat.
2. 2.Add onion and garlic and cook for about 5 mins.
3. Once soft, add salt, ginger, turmeric powder, water, and broccoli florets. Add what is left of the cocnut milk.
4. 4.Let it simmer for 5mins, stir continuously to mash the broccoli
5. 5.Let the mixture cool and pour it into a food processor to blend.
6. To be served with roasted almonds, yogurt, sesame seeds, and fresh greens

Time: 15 minutes

Amount:4 servings

Calories: 250kcal

Carbs: 5.6g

Protein:7.1g

Fat: 21.7g

INGREDIENTS

- Riced cauliflower (3 cups)
- Shredded Asiago cheese (1 cup)
- Heavy cream (3/4 cup)
- Fresh basil (chopped, optional)

HOW TO COOK

1. Add riced cauliflower into a saute pan. Add 2 tbsp of water, cover then cook for about 5 minutes

2. Add cheese and cream and mix until cheese melts

3. Taste to see if cauliflower is ready

4. Remove from heat and serve. You can add freshly chopped basil to top

Time: 25 minutes

Amount:3 servings

Calories: 263 kcal

Carbs: 5g

Protein:27g

Fat: 13g

INGREDIENTS

- Chicken breasts (10 oz/1.2kg)-boneless
- 2 tablespoon Worcestershire sauce
- ½ tablespoon Onion powder
- ½ tablespoon Garlic powder
- Dash ground pepper

- 2 tablespoons Olive oil
- ½ cup frozen or fresh onion
- ½ tablespoon minced garlic
- 3 slices of Provolone cheese
- ½ cup diced bell pepper
- 10 oz boneless chicken breasts (2)

HOW TO COOK

1. 1.Set the chicken breast in a bowl after cutting it into thin slices.

2. Add ground pepper, Worcestershire sauce, onion poweder, garlic powder, and ground pepper. Stir till the chicken is completely coated.

3. In a skillet, heat 1 tablespoon oil and add the chicken pieces. Cook for 5mins till the color turns brown. Cook for 3mins on each side till its brown and remove from the skillet.

4. 4.Add onion, bell pepper, garlic, and olive oil to the skillet. Cook and stir for about 3mins till it is tender.

5. 5.Reduce the heat and return chicken to the skillet, add veggies and stir to mix properly. Add in the sliced cheese and cover skillet for about 3 minutes until cheese melts

Time: 25 minutes

Amount:2 servings

Calories: 575

Carbohydrates: 7g

Protein: 20g

Fat: 51g

INGREDIENTS

- Avocado (1, medium)
- Eggs (6)
- ½ tablespoon chopped parsley
- Add salt and peper to taste
- 1 tablespoon Dijon Mustard
- 1/3 cup Mayonnaise
- A splash of Lemon juice (keeps avocado from browning)
- Dill (1/8 tsp)

HOW TO MAKE

1. Boil eggs in a saucepan. Cover the pan and let it cool for 15mins.

2. Run under cold water then peel the shells off

3. Chop eggs into pieces, add pepper, salt and set it aside. Repeat the process with the avocado.

4. Mix the mayo, eggs, and the mashed avocado along with lemon juice, mustard and any herbs of choice

5. Serve chilled\

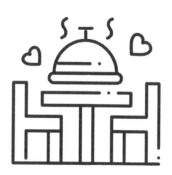

Time: 20 minutes

Amount:3 servings

Calories: 325kcal

Carbs: 3g

Protein: 39g

Fat: 16g

INGREDIENTS

- Shirataki angel hair noodles (2 packs 7oz/200g)
- Pastured chicken breast (1 lb/0.45kg)
- Cooking oil (1 tablespoon)
- Organic garlic (1 large, minced)
- Dried oregano (1/2 tsp) or fresh oregano leaves (1 tsp, minced)
- ½ tablespoon Himalayan pink salt
- Lemon juice from one large lemon kept separate and lemon zest
- Butter or grass-fed ghee
- Collagelatin (1 tbsp)
- Fresh oregano leaves (1 to 2 tbsp)

HOW TO COOK

1. To cook the shirataki noodles, follow package guide and directions. Set aside after cooking.

2. Over medium-high heat, heat the skillet then add oil.

3. 3.Add dried oregano, dried oregano, chicken, garlic, and salt to the skillet and cook for 10mins till it is fully cooked. Cook and stir for 10mins. Set aside after removing the chicken.

4. Reduce the heat with the skillet still on and add lemon juice. Next, add in the butter then stir until it melts. Whisk in the collagelatin

5. Return chicken and noodles to skillet. Toss to combine

6. To be served with lemon zest as a topping and garnished with fresh oregano

Time:30 minutes

Amount: 4 servings

Calories 406

Carbohydrates 8g

Protein 28g

Fat 29g

INGREDIENTS

- Cut 1 lb/0.45kg chicken breasts into smaller bite-sized pieces.
- 1 ½ cupbok choy cleanedand sliced
- ½ cup Rawcashew pieces
- ½ cup Stalkscelery (thinly sliced)
- ½ cup Canned full-fat Coconutmilk
- 2 tablespoon Coconut Aminos
- 2 tablespoon Garlic powder
- 1/3 cup Shallot
- ¼ cup Coconut oil
- Add salt and pepper to taste
- ½ cup Fresh chopped cilantro

HOW TO COOK

1. In a large skillet, melt oil then add in the shallots, garlic, and celery. Saute till the shallot becomes until the shallots becomes lucid

2. Add chicken. Cook until it is browned then add in cashews, garlic powder, bok choy, and coconut milk.

3. Cook until the meat is well cooked and the coconut milk as reduce to a glaze.

4. Remove skillet from heat then toss in fresh cilantro and coconut aminos.

5. 5.Add salt and pepper and serve.

Time: 30minutes

Amount:11 servings

Calories: 268kcal

Carbs: 10g

Protein 41g

Fat: 7.5g

INGREDIENTS

- Chicken breasts (1.5lbs/0.7kg)
- Add Kosher salt to taste
- ½ cup low sodium chicken broth
- 2 tablespoons Low sodium shoyu or coconut amino
- 2 tablespoons Water
- Cornstarch or arrow root powder or tapioca starch (2 teaspoon)
- Grapeseed oil (1 tbsp) or canola
- Asparagus (1 bunch), ends cut and trimmed to pieces (2-inches)
- Garlic (6 cloves)
- 3 tablespoons Fresh lemon juice
- Add fresh black pepper to taste
- 1 tablespoon fresh ginger

HOW TO COOK

1. Season chicken lightly with salt.

2. In a bowl, mix the soy sauce and chicken sauce.

3. Mix corn starch in a separate bowl and add water to mix better.

4. Heat a non-stick wok over medium to high heat. Add 1tbsp oil and asparagus. Let it cook for 3mins till crisp and tender.

5. Add ginger and garlic. Cook for 1min till color turns golden. Remove then set aside.

6. Set the heat at high and add 1 tablespoon of oil. In the oil, cook the chicken in half for 4mins till browned and cooked through on each side.

7. Remove chicken and set aside. Repeat this process for the entire chicken and set aside.

8. Cook for 2mins and add soy sauce.

9. Add cornstarch and lemon juice mixture. Stir when then return the asparagus and chicken earlier set aside.

10. Separate the work from the heat and mix.

Time: 17 minutes

Amount:4 servings

Calories: 319kcal

Carbs: 11g,

Protein: 18g

Fat: 24g

INGREDIENTS

For Shrimp

- Extra-large shrimp (1lbs/0.45kg), peeled & deveined
- 1 tablespoon butter

- 1 tablespoon Olive oil
- Black pepper
- Salt

For Salad

- Cucumber (1 ½ cups)
- Chopped Red onions (1 cup)
- 1 cup chopped red bell pepper
- Avocado (2 medium, peeled, chopped and pitted)

- 2 tablespoons Lemon juice
- Chopped parsley
- 4 tablespoons Olive oil
- Black pepper
- Salt

HOW TO COOK

1. Pat dry shrimp with paper towels
2. Over medium-high heat, heat the butter and olive oil in a skillet. Add the shrimpsthen add salt and pepper
3. On each side, cook for about 2mins until it is cooked through.
4. In a salad bowl, add cucumber, bell pepper, avocado, red onions, and the shrimp.
5. Pour salt, lemon juice, olive oil, and black pepper in a mason jar. Mix seasoning and taste then pour over salad.
6. Toss salad and serve

Time: 30 minutes

Amount:4 servings

Calories: 319kcal

Carbs: 11g,

Protein: 18g

Fat: 24g

Ingredients

- Fajitas Seasoning Mix (Homemade)
- Olive oil (1 tsp, divided)
- Cut 3 colored bell peppers into thin strips
- Yellow onion (1 large) sliced
- Lime juice (from 1 lime)
- Freshly chopped parsley (or cilantro)
- Guacamole (optional, for serving)

HOW TO COOK

1. Prepare Fajitas seasoning and set it aside
2. Cut steak into strips about 6" long and 2" wide
3. Rub strips with prepared seasoning then set aside
4. Place a grill pan over medium-high heat and heat the oil. Add sliced onions and pepper strips. To season, add pepper and salt. You can also sprinkle some of the fajitas seasonings as well.
5. 5.To make it tender, cook for about 5mins. Set aside after removing from the heat to cool.
6. Each steak slice should be topped with vegetables. Roll it up and use a toothpick to secure it.
7. Add olive oil to grill pan and heat it then add the roll-ups to the pan.
8. Cooked on each side for about 3mins
9. Remove from heat. Transfer to serving plate after removing the toothpicks.
10. Squeeze some lime juice over roll-ups and garnish as preferred.

Time: 20 minutes

Amount:4 servings

Calories: 411.1kcal

Carbs: 11.7g,

Protein: 45.7g

Fat 18.8g

INGREDIENTS

- ◆ 1 medium diced onion
- ◆ 450-500 chicken fillets
- ◆ ½ tablespoon coconut butter
- ◆ Two medium zucchinis
- ◆ 400g crushed tomato
- ◆ 100g raw cashews
- ◆ 7-10 cherry tomato chopped in half
- ◆ Salt, dry oregano, pepper, and basil for seasoning

HOW TO COOK

1. Place a pan over high-medium heat and heat it. Add onions and cocnut butter and cook for about 1min. Cook careful to prevent the onions from getting burnt.

2. Dice the chicken and make it into 2cm.

3. To the heated pan, add garlic and chicken. Season with dried basil, salt, ground black pepper, and oregano. Let the chicken cook for about 6 mins or till its golden.

4. Spiralizer the zucchini. Use a vegei peeler in the absence of a spiralizer. Use it to make ribbons out of it and cut the zucchini shorter when you need to.

5. Add crushed tomato to the golden chicken and wait to simmer for about 5mins.

6. In a separate pan, roast the raw cashew till it appears golden. Use salt, ground turmeric, and paprika as seasoning.

7. Add cherry tomato, spiralized zoodles, and salt as season when needed. You might need to cut the zoodles shorter when they are too long. Cook for 1 minute and switch off the oven.

8. Serve with fresh basil leaves or spiced cashews.

Time: 1hr 30 minutes

Amount:8 servings

Calories: 422kcal

Carbs: 4g.

Protein: 24g

Fat 24g

INGREDIENTS

- 1 tablespoon Dried tarragon
- Chicken (500g, minced)
- 1 tablespoon extra-virgin oil
- 1 leek, trimmed, thinly sliced
- 200g sliced button mushroom (punnet)
- Chopped and dried English spinach (1 bunch)
- 250g chopped packet cream cheese
- Tomato pasta sauce (125ml, ½ cup)
- 40g (1/2) parmesan (finely grated)
- 1 cup 100g mozzarella (coarsely grated)
- **Cauliflower Lasagne Sheets**
- 2eggs
- trimmed or coarsely chopped cauliflower

HOW TO COOK

1. Process1/2 of the cauliflower for the lasagne sheet in a food processor till it is finely chopped. Move it to a microwave bowl.

2. Go over this process for the cauliflower that is left. Microwave on high and stir occasionally for about 10mins till it is very tender.

3. Use a fine sieve to drain and use a wooden spoon to press down to get rid of excess water. Add egg and parmesan and stir well with seasoning to mix.

4. Set oven at 160 °C or 180 °C an-forced. Use baking paper to line the baking trays. Split the cauliflower mixture into the two trays and use a palette knife or your fingertip to press it into a rectangle of 22*30 cm.

5. Let it cook till the mixture dries out and let it cool at a side. Cut it into about 6 lasagna sheets 10cm wide each.

6. Use a non-stick frying pan to heat the oil over high heat. Reduce the heat and add leek. Stirr often for about 4mins till it softens.

7. Revert the heat to hhigh and add the chicken. Cook for about 5mins, breaking it up with a wooden spoon till the msurooms appear golden.

8. Cook and stir for 4mins occasional after adding the spinach till it is wilted. Add spinach. Add cream cheese. Stir and cook for 2mins till the chesses melts. Set aside after stiring through the season and the tarragon.

9. Grease the baking dish and use a tomato pasta sauce to lightly brush the base of the dish. The measurement should be 24cm (top measurement) 19cm (base measurement) Use ½ of the chicken mixture and 1/3 cup sprinkle mozzarella as topping.

10. Do this process again with the chicken mixture and cauliflower layer that is left. Use the lasagne left as topping. Conclude this process with the mozzarella and pasta sauce that is left.

11. Let it bake for about 30mins or till a golden color appears. Let it cool for 7mins and serve.

Time: 30 minutes

Amount:4-6 servings

Calories: 487.7kcal

Carbs: 7.3g

Protein 33.8g

Fat 35.8g

INGREDIENTS

- 1 ½ pounds boneless skinless chicken breasts, thinly sliced
- 2 tablespoons olive oil
- 1 cup heavy cream
- ½ cup chicken broth
- 1 teaspoon garlic powder
- Parmesan cheese (1/2 cup)
- Chopped spinach (1 cup)
- Sun-dried tomatoes (½ cup)
- 1 tablespoon Italian seasoning

HOW TO COOK

1. Add sufficient amount of olive oil to a large skillet. On high-medium heat, cook the chicken for about 5mins till it browns on each side or you till the pink center is no longer visible.

2. Prepare a separate plate and set the chicken aside after removing it from the skillet.

3. Add the chicken broth, garlic powder, heavy cream, parmesan cheese, and Italian seasoning. To make it thicken, whisk it over medium-high heat.

4. Add sundried tomatoes and spinach, let it simmer to make the spinach wilt.

5. Return the chicken to the pan and add pastea to serving if you want.

Time: 30minutes

Amount:4 servings

Calories: 151.6kcal

Carbs: 3.4g

Protein 30g

Fat 2g

INGREDIENTS

- 1.2kg chicken Marylands (4)
- 15g butter
- Extra-virgin olive oil (1 tbsp)
- 80ml (1/3) Massel salt, chicken style stock (liquid)
- 1 large red onion, halved, cut into thin wedges
- 80ml white wine (1/3, dry)
- 300g (2 cups) frozen broad beans
- 80ml (1/3 cup) pouring cream
- 1/3 cup fresh tarragon leaves, plus extra, to serve

HOW TO COOK

1. Set oven to 180°C for 200C fan-forced. In a large oven, heat ½ of the oil in a pan over medium heat. Season the chicken. Cook, the chicken for about 5mins with the side down till it turns golden. Pour to a new plate to get rid of the fat.

2. Over a low-medium heat, heat the butter that is left. Cook onion and turn continuously until it turns golden. Add the wine. Simmer for 1 minute. Add stock. Simmer for 1 minute. Remove the heat.

3. Bake for about 30mins with the onion below the chicken till it is cooked through. Use a baking paper to line the tray. Transfer chicken to prepared tray and keep it warm by sending it back in the oven.

4. Meanwhile, place the broad beans in a heatproof bowl. For 2mins, cover it and drain. Drain. Use cold water to refresh and peel.

5. Return to medium heat. Let it simmer for about 2mins till it is slightly reduced. Add a cream and cream and leave to simmer for about 3mins until it thickens. Add the tarragon. Simmer for 1 minute. Remove chicken to the pan. Sprinkle with remaining broad beans and extra tarragon.

6. Serve with 1 chopped avocado and mixed salad leaves to increase the ratio of fat to protein and carbs.

Time: 20minutes

Amount:4 servings

Calories: 230kcal

Carbs: 11g

Protein 30g

Fat 9g

INGREDIENTS

- 1 tablespoon salt, divided
- Cut 1 pounder turkey tenderloin to about 1/4-inch-thick thin steaks
- ½ large sliced sweet onion
- Ground black pepper (1/2 tbsp)
- Extra-virgin olive oil (2tbsp)
- Cut 1 red bell pepper into strips
- Red wine (2 tbsp vinegar)
- Cut 1 yellow bell pepper into strips
- Basil and chopped fresh parsley for garnish though optional
- 114-ounce can-crushed tomatoes, preferably fine-roasted

HOW TO COOK

1. Over the turkey, add ½ tsp salt. In a skillet, add 1 tbsp oil and heat over high-medium heat.

2. Cook after adding half turkey till the bottom becomes brown. Flip continuously for about 2mins till it beomes brown.

3. Transfer the turkey with a slotted spatula to a plate and keep it warm with a tent foil. Add the remaining 1 tablespoon oil to the skillet. Turn down the heat and repeat the process for about 3mins per side for the turkey left.

4. Add bell peppers, ½ tsp salt, and onion to the skillet. Cover and cook. Stir continuously for about 7mins till the peppers and onions are softened or browned.

5. Turn up the heat to high-medium heat and sprinkle with pepper and Italian seasoning. Cook and stir continuously for about 30secons til the herbs are fragrant.

6. Cook with vinegar and stir continuously til it almost evaporates. Let it simmer and add tomatoes. Stir contiosly.

7. Add to the skillet the accumulated juices and the turkey. Reduce the heat to low-medium heat and let it simmer. Cook and turn the sauce continiosuly till the turkey is hot. Do this for about 2mins and serve when it is done with basil and parsley as toppings.

Time: 45minutes

Amount:4 servings

Calories: 684.496kcal

Carbs: 7g

Protein 32g

Fat 57g

INGREDIENTS

- ½ teaspoon turmeric
- Fresh ginger (2 tsps, finely grated)
- Cut 600g chicken thigh fillets into pieces (3cm)
- Macadamia oil (2tbsp)
- Red chilies, finely chopped (2 long)
- 1 Brown sliced onion
- 2 crushed garlic cloves
- 2 teaspoons brown mustard seeds
- 1 teaspoon ground coriander
- 400ml can coconut cream
- 500g broccoli, chopped
- Limejuice
- Fish sauce, to taste
- 100g baby spinach leaves

HOW TO COOK

1. Prepare a saucepan and heat oil over high heat. Use only half the oil.

2. Cook half the chicken and stir continuously fr about 3mins till it is brown.

3. Set a new pan and add the oil that is left and onion. Cook and stir for another 4mins till it softens.

4. Add the ginger, mustard seed, chili, turmeric, cumin, coriander, and garlic. Stir and cook for about 2mins and add the chicken and coconut cream.

5. Cover the pan halfway and turn down the heat. Let it simmer for about 20 minutes till the chicken becomes tender.

6. Put in the broccoli in batches in a food processor till it is finely chopped to look like rice.

7. Move the broccoli to a prepared microwave bowl. Cover the safe bowl and leave it high for about 3mins till it is tender.

8. Use fish sauce and lime juice as season and get rid of the curry. Sprinkle with extra chilli and spinach to serve with broccoli rice.

Time: 20minutes

Amount:4 servings

Calories: 285kcal

Carbs: 1.4g

Protein 27.8g

Fat 18.9g

INGREDIENTS

- ◆ Crème Fraiche (3 tbsp)
- ◆ 250g smoked salmon (sliced)
- ◆ large eggs (6, beaten)
- ◆ Chopped chives (1 tbsp)
- ◆ Black pepper and salt
- ◆ horseradish sauce (1 tbsp)
- ◆ Lemon juice
- ◆ Salad leaves to serve

HOW TO COOK

1. Set the oven to 160° C to 180° C fan-forced. Use little oil to grease the ramekins. Ine the ramekin with smoked salmon on the inside with no gaps left but with enough room over the edges. Use the edge to cover the top when you are done.

2. Line the remaining salmon and cut it into small chumps. Add the beaton egg and chives. Season with black pepper and salt.

3. After lining the ramekins, pour in the egg mixture and fold it over the salmon

4. Prepare a baking tray and place the ramekins on it. Pour 5cm water deep water into the tray and let it bake for about 20mins in the oven till it is firm to touch.

5. Mix the black pepper, lemon juice, horseradish, and crème Fraiche.

6. After cooking the egg, turn upside down on a plate after removing the water. Remove the ramekin and serve with salad leaves and hollandaise.

Time: 20minutes

Amount:4 servings

Calories: 388kcal

Carbs: 9.3g

Protein 30g

Fat 29g

INGREDIENTS

Broccoli

- Fine salt (1/2 tbsp)
- Avocado oil (1 tbsp)
- Cut 4 broccoli crowns into florets

Beef

- Cooking fat (1 tbsp)
- Granulated garlic (1tbsp)
- Fine salt (1 tbsp)
- Coconut aminos (1 tbsp)
- Ground beef lean grass fed (1 pound 85%)

Sunshine sauce

- Bone broth (1/4 cup)
- Ground ginger (1 tbsp)
- Ground pepper (1 tsp)
- Sunflower seed butter oil (2 tbsp)
- Cooking fat (1 tbsp)
- Coconut aminos (2 tbsp)
- Lemon juice
- 1 Mined green onion
- Fine salt (1/2)

Assembling

- Baby spinach (4 cups) though optional

HOW TO COOK

1. Set oven at 400 ° F. Prepare a sheet pan and mix the salt and fat with the broccoli. Spread the fat by massaging it into the florets and spread them on the sheet to prevent overcrowding.

2. While the oven pre-heats, put in the sheet pan and set the timer at 20mins.

3. Over medium heat, heat a skillet and add the fat when the temperature is reached.

4. Add garlic and salt to the skiller and crumble gound beef in it. Stir continuously and whisk till it is crumbly or browned. Increase the heat and put coconut aminos.

5. Cook and stir continuously till crispy or dark brown.

6. In the meanwhile, set a small saucepot over medium heat.

7. Melt the fat than the sunflower seed, stirring until smooth.

8. Addd the ground ginger, salt aminos, and bone broth. Stir continuously till it mixes well.

9. Set down from the heat and add lemon juice. Stir till it is smooth.

10. Mix in the green onions. Set aside.

11. In a bowl, make a bed of 4 large baby spinach. In the bowl, add the ground beef and broccoli florets. To complete the assembling, spoon the sauce over it.

Time: 20minutes

Amount:6 servings

Calories: 427kcal

Carbs: 2.2g

Protein 8.7g

Fat 34g

INGREDIENTS

- Avocado, peeled, sliced (1 large)
- 175g shortcut bacon rasher
- Cut 1 medium tomato into wedges
- A teaspoon American mustard
- 2 Green onions, thinly sliced
- White wine vinegar (2 tsp)
- Olive oil (2 tbsp)

HOW TO COOK

1. Let the frying pan heat over memdium heat.
2. Let the bacon cook for about 2mins till it is lighly browned on each side. Roughly chop, transfer to a bowl.
3. Add avocado, onion, and tomato.
4. Place mustard, oil, and vinegar in a jug.
5. Whisk to combine. Combine and toss it with salad.

Time: 25minutes

Servings:2 servings

Calories: 301kcal

Carbs: 8.3g

Protein 32.7g

Fat 15.2g

INGREDIENTS

- 1 pound extra-lean ground beef
- 9-ounce bag coleslaw mix, purple cabbage, carrot, and shredded cabbage.
- Sesame oil (1tbsp)
- Rice vinegar (2 tablespoons)
- Garlic, minced (2 cloves)
- ¼ tbsp red pepper flakes
- Soy sauce ¼ cup (to replace soy, use coconut aminos, tamari, or wheat)
- ½ tablespoon salt
- Scallions for garnish (Chopped, optional)
- Grated fresh ginger (1tbsp)
- ¼ tablespoon ground black pepper

HOW TO COOK

1. In a small bowl, combine the rice vinegar, soy sauce, black pepper, red pepper falkes, and salt.
2. Prepare a large skillet and heat the sesame oil over high-medium heat. Include the beef and let it cook for about b9 mins till it is browned.
3. Add ginger and garlic and cook for about 2mins.
4. Mix the soy sauce and coleslaw mix into the skiller. Let it cook for about 7mins. Stir to soften the cabbage.
5. Use chopped scallions as garnish.

SNACKS AND DESSERT RECIPES

Time: 2hrs 30 mins – 3hrs

Amount: 16 servings

Calories: 254.19 kcal

Protein: 7.9g

Fat: 23.4g

Net carb: 2.49g

INGREDIENTS

- ½ teaspoon of lemon
- Vanilla extract (1 ½ teaspoons)
- Salt ½ teaspoon
- Softened unsalted butter (1/2 cup)
- Almond flour (2 ½ cups)
- 8 eggs
- Erythritol (1 ½ cups)
- Cream cheese (8 oz)
- 1 ½ teaspoons. baking powder
- **Glaze**
- Vanilla extract (1/2 tsp)
- ¼ cup powdered erythritol
- 3 teaspoons Softened beating cream

HOW TO COOK

1. Preheat oven to 3500F. In a mixing bowl, mix butter, softened cream cheese, and erythritol at room temperature.

2. Continue the mixing in the bowl until the butter and erythritol becomes smooth. Bring in the chunks of cream cheese, and blend till smooth.

3. Add in eggs; and the extract of lemon and vanilla into the blended ingredients. Use a hand mixer to blend till smooth.

4. Mix baking powder, almond flour, and salt in a small bowl.

5. Gently add the mixture of the almond flour, powder, and salt into the batter. Again, use a hand blender to blend the clumps until smooth.

6. Get a loaf pan and pour the batter into it. Bake at 350°F for 60-120mins or bake until the middle is smooth.

7. For a glaze, pour the vanilla extract, powdered erythritol, and heavy beating cream in a blender; and blend until smooth. Ensure that the cake gets cool in the oven before spreading the glaze.

Time: 23 minutes

Serving: 8-12 cookies

Calories: 113 kcal

Fat: 18.8g

Protein: 1g

INGREDIENTS

- ◆ 1 cup unsweetened shredded coconut
- ◆ 1 tablespoon almond meal or flour of choice
- ◆ ½ cup plus 1 tablespoon milk of choice or coconut milk
- ◆ 1/16 teaspoon salt
- ◆ 3 ½ tablespoons pure maple syrup, honey, or agave
- ◆ ¼ teaspoon pure vanilla or coconut extract

HOW TO COOK

1. Allow the oven heat up to 350ºF, then arrange your baking tins/dish with a silicone mat or parchment paper.

2. Place a cup of coconut in the oven for about 8-10mins.

3. Take out the toasted coconut and pour into a large bowl. Mix with all other ingredients.

4. Prepare a baking sheet and place a tablespoon round cookie scoops on it.

5. Put the baking sheet into the oven to bake for 18-20 mins.

6. Allow ½ cup of dark vegan chocolate to melt completely. Remove the cookies from the oven and allow it to cooldown. Dip the bottom of the cookies into the melted chocolate and place them on a parchment paper. Place it in a fridge for 5-10mins. You do not need to refrigerate it if you don't dip the cookies into the chocolate.

7. Serve yourself a sumptuous dish. You can also add your favourite non-dairy milk to enjoy

Time: 34 minutes

Amount: 20 keto double chocolate chip cookies

Calories: 106 kcal

Fat: 9g

Protein: 5g

Carb: 2g

INGREDIENTS

- 1 ¼ cup nut butter or almond butter
- 2 eggs
- ½ cup of cocoa powder
- 1 teaspoon of baking powder.
- ½ cup powdered low-carb sweetener, to taste
- Salt (if nut butter isn't already salted)
- ¼ cup dark chocolate chunks

HOW TO COOK

1. Preheat oven to 350ºF

2. Mix all ingredient with a hand mixer, in a large bowl with the exemption of the chocolate chunks.

3. Fold chocolate chunks

4. Scoop out dough and place on a baking pan that is lined with parchment paper.

5. Place in oven for 12-14 mins.

6. After baking, take the cookies out of the oven and place on a baking rack. Let it cool for 15 mins then serve and enjoy.

Time: 20 minutes

Amount: 10 servings

Calories: 202 kcal

Fat: 18.6g

Carbohydrates: 4.4g

Protein: 1.7g

INGREDIENTS

- 12-ounces strawberries
- Full-fat sour cream (1½ cups)
- Vanilla extract (1 teaspoon)
- 1 ½ cups of heavy cream
- ½ cup powdered swerve sweetener divided

HOW TO COOK

1. Place the strawberries and ¼ of the sweetener in a blender. Blend until almost pureed but some chunks remain.

2. Whisk the vanilla extract, sour cream, and strawberry mixture in a large bowl. Whisk until thoroughly combined.

3. Take another large bowl and whip the leftover ¼ cup sweetener with cream until it holds stiff peaks. Pour the whipped cream into the strawberry mixture until just a few streaks remain.

4. Pour into a container and put in the fridge until firm. It can take up to 6 hours to freeze.

Time: 40 minutes

Yield: 8 servings

Calories: 152kcal

Fat: 13.8g

Carbohydrates: 10g

Protein: 3.9g

INGREDIENTS

- 2 eggs
- ¼ cup lard or coconut oil (melted ghee)
- 1/3 cup cacao powder
- 1 avocado (medium and ripe)
- Salt (1/4 teaspoon)
- Granulated sweetener (xylitol, coconut palm, maple sugar) or 1/3 cup erythritol + monk fruit
- 3-4 tablespoons almond butter (unsweetened), cashew butter or sunflower seed butter for nut-free
- 1 tsp vanilla extract
- ½ teaspoon baking soda
- Gelatine (2 tbsps.)
- ½ cup low carb chocolate chips

HOW TO COOK

1. Pre-heat oven to 350ºF

2. Line a loaf pan with parchment paper.

3. Combine all ingredients in a blender.

4. Blend the ingredients with medium, low power until smooth. This takes about half a minute. It can be cakey if mixed for too long. With the use of a spatula, scrape the mixture and fold it together, mashing up any chunk of avocado left.

5. Transfer the batter to a baking dish still with the spatula, and smooth it out evenly.

6. You can spread fun things on it, for topping.

7. Put the baking dish in the oven and allow to bake for about 25 mins or until the edges begin to separate from the sides.

8. Once done, take it from the oven and allow to cool for 15 mins.

9. Pick it up by the parchment paper and place on a cutting board.

10. You can cut out 8 squares from it. Enjoy! You can also keep leftovers in the fridge for up to 7 days.

Time: 10 minutes

Serving: 4 chocolate mousse

Calories: 239kcal

Carbs: 2g

Fat: 22g

Protein: 3g

Fiber: 4g

INGREDIENTS

- 1.76oz dark chocolate
- 0.53oz salted butter or unsalted butter + pinch of salt
- 1 tbsp cocoa powder
- 6.76floz whipping cream
- Stevia to taste

HOW TO COOK

1. Put the chocolate and butter in a microwave, to melt for 30 seconds, then mix.
2. Whip together cream, cocoa powder, and stevia
3. Add in the chocolate and butter mix
4. Whip till soft peaks are formed and put into bowls
5. Refrigerate for 1 hour at least and serve cold

Time: 25 minutes

Serving: 12 donuts

Fat: 10g

Saturated fat: 3g

Carbohydrate: 3g

Calories: 110kcal

Protein: 3g

INGREDIENTS

- ¼ almond milk (unsweetened)
- ¼ cup powdered monk fruit sweetener
- Xanthan gum (1/4 teaspoon)
- 2 eggs
- Vanilla extract (1 teaspoon)
- Coconut flour (1/2 tablespoon)
- Pumpkin pie spice (1 teaspoon)
- Ground cinnamon (½ teaspoon)
- Baking powder (1 ½ teaspoons)
- Baking soda (1/2 teaspoon)
- Salt
- Sugar-fine lightened almond flour (1 cup)
- 2 tablespoons Melted ghee or butter (if not paleo)
- 2 tablespoons pure pumpkin puree
- Mini donut pan
- **Topping**
- **To coat the pumpkin with spice**
- Pumpkin pie spice (1 teaspoon)
- Melted ghee (1 ½ tablespoons)
- ¼ cup granulated monk fruit sweetener

HOW TO COOK

1. Whisk almond milk, egg, melted ghee, pumpkin puree, vanilla, and monk fruit sweetener in a large bowl until smooth and combined.

2. Mix the almond flour, xanthan gum, coconut flour, cinnamon, pumpkin pie spice, baking soda, baking powder, and salt in a medium bowl. Add the mixed dry ingredients slowly into the mixed wet ingredients; and stir until combined.

3. Pour the batter into a greased 12 cavity silicone donut pan or mini muffin tins (filling ¾ full). For regular size donuts, you can use a 6-cavity silicone donut pan

4. Preheat oven to 350°F, then put the donut pan into the oven to bake for 12-15 mins (for min) or 21-24 mins (for regular size) until golden brown.

5. Remove the donuts from the oven when well baked, and allow to cool

For the pumpkin spice coating

6. Stir the granulated sweetener and pumpkin pie spice in a small bowl while the donuts are still in the oven.

7. Melt ghee or butter in a separate small bowl

8. Dunk each donut in melted ghee and roll into the cinnamon/sweetener coating.

9. Repeat with remaining donuts.

Time: 20 minutes

Serving: 4 servings

Calories: 258kcal

Fat: 25g

Carbohydrate: 2g

Protein: 7g

INGREDIENTS

- 4 lemons (juice and zest)
- ½ cup Natvia or erythritol
- 100g butter
- 3 whole eggs
- 1 egg yolk

HOW TO COOK

1. Grab a medium heatproof bowl and squeezer the lemons, zest the skin, add the natvia (or erythritol) and add the butter.

2. Place the bowl over a pan of boiling water. Avoid touching the bottom of the pan with the bowl. Then begin to until the butter melts.

3. Lightly whisk the eggs and egg yolk, then stir into the heated mixture. Continue stirring for 10 mins till the back of the spoon becomes coated.

4. Take it from the heat and pour into sterilized jars. You can store it in a fridge for 2 weeks.

Losing 11 pounds in 3 weeks can be a daunting task. A task that not so many diet plans can help achieve. Interestingly, one diet plan that offers faster weight loss results is the keto diet. By activating ketosis, it forces the body to empty its fat stores for energy.

To make growth effective, it must be deliberate and planned. However, you should make it a point to always remember that the plan is not rigid but can be adjusted to suit your environment and preference. To make it easy, a meal plan will help you through this journey as it will teach you how to switch between meals to maintain your health.

This is an eating plan for 21 days and it is designed exclusively to get you through your weight loss journey.

DAY 1

Breakfast : Bulletproof coffee egg latte
(Serves 1/12 minutes) (page 18)

Calories: 331Kcal

Carbs: 4.5g

Protein: 24g

Fat: 25g

INGREDIENTS

- Black coffee (8 oz/227g)
- Grass-fed butter or ghee (1 to 2 tbsp)
- Brain octane oil (1 to 2 tbsp)
- Pastured raised egg-2 eggs
- Vanilla collagen protein (1 scoop)
- Ceylon Cinnamon (1/4 teaspoon)

HOW TO COOK

1. Blend eggs, oil, butter, and cinnamon until well mixed
2. Add coffee then blend for 45 seconds more on high speed
3. To this, add the collagen protein then blend for 5 more seconds at low speed
4. Add cinnamon for topping

Lunch : Loaded chicken salad (page 36)

Dinner : Low-Carb Angel Hair Pasta With Lemon Chicken (page 52)

DAY 2

Breakfast: Fluffy almond flour paleo pancakes (page 19)
Lunch : Zucchini crust grilled cheese (serves: 2/40 mins) (page 37)

Calories: 155kcal

Carbs: 5g

Protein: 10g

Fat: 10g

INGREDIENTS

- Shredded zucchini (4 cups)
- 1 egg
- ½ cup shredded Mozzarella cheese
- 4 tablespoons grated Parmesan cheese
- ½ tablespoon salt
- A pinch pepper (black)
- 1 tablespoon dried Oregano
- **For Grilled cheese**
- Room temperature butter
- Cheddar cheese (grated or shredded) 1/3 cup

HOW TO COOK

1. Preheat the oven to 450°F or 220°C. Prepare a baking sheet by lining with parchment paper and greasing it

2. Place zucchini in a microwave-safe dish and cook in microwave on high for about 6 minutes. Transfer to a tea towel or dishcloth then twist to get the moisture out. The zucchini should be as dry as possible otherwise you end up with a mushy dough

3. Mix zucchini with egg, Parmesan cheese, salt, oregano, mozzarella cheese, and pepper. Spread this mixture on the lined sheet then shape into 4 square.

4. Bake in preheated oven for 15-20 minutes

5. Remove from oven then leave to cool for about 10 minutes before peeling it carefully off the parchment sheet.

6. Heat pan over medium heat, butter each slice of zucchini crusty bread on one side. Place the slice in a pan with the buttered side below, sprinkle with cheese then top with the remaining slice of bread with the buttered side up.

7. Turn heat down slightly then cook for about 2 to 4 minutes until color turns golden brown. Flip gently and cook the other side for another 2-4 minutes.

Dinner : Bok Choy Chicken Stir Fry (page 53)

DAY 3

Breakfast : Coconut flour crepes (page 20)

Lunch : Easy shrimp avocado salad with tomatoes and feta (page 38)

Dinner: Chicken and asparagus lemon stir fry (Serves 11/30 minutes) (page 54)

Calories: 268kcal

Carbs: 10g

Protein 41g

Fat: 7.5g

INGREDIENTS

- Chicken breasts (1.5lbs/0.7kg)
- Kosher salt (added to taste)
- Low sodium chicken broth (1/2 cup)
- Low sodium shoyu or coconut amino (2 tbsp)
- Water (2 tbsp)
- Cornstarch or tapioca starch or arrowroot powder (2 tsp)
- Grapeseed oil (1 tbsp) or canola
- Asparagus (1 bunch), ends trimmed and cut into pieces (2-inches)
- Garlic (6 cloves)
- Fresh lemon juice (3 tbsp)
- Fresh black pepper (added to taste)
- Fresh ginger (1 tbsp)

HOW TO COOK

1. Season chicken lightly with salt.
2. Mix chicken broth and soy sauce in a small bowl
3. In another bowl, mix cornstarch with water then mix well
4. Heat a non-stick wok over medium to high heat. Add 1 teaspoon of oil then add asparagus and cook for about 3 minutes till tender and crisp.
5. Add ginger and garlic then cook for about a minute until color turns golden. Remove then set aside.
6. Turn the heat to high and add 1 tsp of oil. Cook half of the chicken in oil (about 4 minutes on each side) till browned and cooked through.
7. Remove chicken and set aside. Do this for the remaining chicken using the rest of the oil. Set aside when done.

8. Add soy sauce mixture boil and cook for 1 to 2 minutes.

9. Add cornstarch and lemon juice mixture. Stir when then return the asparagus and chicken earlier set aside.

10. Mix well, remove the wok from the heat then serve.

DAY 4

Breakfast: Collagen keto bread (serves 12/1hr 50 minutes) (page 21)

Carbs: 1g

Protein: 7g

Fat: 5g

INGREDIENTS

- Collagen Protein-Unflavored, Grass-Fed (1/2 cup)
- Almond flour
- Pastured eggs (5, separated)
- Unflavored coconut oil (1 tbsp)
- Baking powder (1 tsp)
- Xanthan gum (1 tsp)
- Himalayan salt
- Stevia (optional)

HOW TO COOK:

1. Oil the bottom of a standard size loaf dish (glass or ceramic). You can use coconut oil, butter or ghee for this or simply lay a piece of parchment paper at the bottom of the dish.

2. Beat egg whites in a large bowl until it begins to form stiff peaks then set aside

3. Mix all dry ingredients in a bowl. Add a pinch of stevia (optional)

4. Whisk wet ingredients in another small bowl

5. Add both dry and wet ingredients to the egg whites. Mix thoroughly until the batter is thick and a bit gooey

6. Pour batter into lined or oiled dish and place in a preheated oven. Bake for 40 minutes.

7. Remove from the oven and leave to cool for about 1 to 2 hours.

8. Remove cooled bread from the baking dish using a knife.

9. Cut into 12 slices and serve

Lunch: Keto chicken enchilada bowl (page 39)

Dinner: Shrimp Avocado Cucumber Salad (page 55)

DAY 5

Breakfast: Keto chocolate cake donuts (page 22)

Lunch: Easy Keto Lasagna Stuffed Portobellos
(Serves 4/60mins) (page 40)

Calories: 482kcal

Carbs: 6.5g

Protein:28g

Fat: 36g

INGREDIENTS

- Portobello mushrooms (4, large)
- Whole milk ricotta cheese
- Italian sausage (4 links)
- Sugar-free marinara sauce (1 cup)
- Mozzarella cheese (shredded)-1 cup
- Chopped parsley (optional, as garnish)

HOW TO COOK

1. Brush portobello mushrooms with a dry paper towel to remove dirt
2. Remove stems and scrape brown ribs with a spoon
3. Remove sausage from casing then press into 4 patties.
4. Press one patty into each of the mushroom caps. Ensure that it goes all the way to the edges and up its sides
5. Spoon some of the ricotta (1/4 cup) into the mushroom cap. Press to the edges. Leave a dent in the center of the cap for the sauce.
6. Spoon some of the marinara sauce (1/4 cup) into each of the mushroom caps on top of the layer of ricotta
7. Sprinkle shredded mozzarella cheese on top of each mushroom (1/4 cup). Place into a preheated oven and bake for 40 minutes.
8. Add parsley to garnish then serve while still hot.

Dinner : Steak fajita roll-ups (page 56)

DAY 6

Breakfast: Low-carb keto donuts (page23)

Lunch: Keto sushi (page 41)

Dinner: Chicken tomato zoodles with spiced cashew (Serves 4/20mins) (page 57)

Calories: 411.1kcal

Carbs: 11.7g,

Protein: 45.7g

Fat 18.8g

INGREDIENTS

- 1 medium diced onion
- 450-500 chicken fillets
- ½ tablespoon coconut butter
- Two medium zucchinis
- 400g crushed tomato
- 100g raw cashews
- 7-10 cherry tomato chopped in half
- Salt, dry oregano, pepper, and basil for seasoning

HOW TO COOK

1. Heat a large pan over medium/high heat. Add coconut butter and onions. Cook for 30 seconds to 1 minute. Be careful not to burn the onions.

2. Slice the chicken into 2 cm pieces.

3. Add the chicken and garlic on a pan. Season with dried basil, oregano, salt, and ground black pepper. Cook chicken for 5-6 minutes or until golden.

4. While the chicken is cooking, spiralizer the zucchini. Cut them shorter when needed. If you don't have a special spiralizer, then just use your vegetable peeler and make ribbons out of zucchini.

5. When the chicken is golden, add crushed tomatoes and let it simmer for 3-5 minutes.

6. While the chicken is cooking, roast the raw cashew in another pan until golden. Season with paprika, salt, and ground turmeric.

7. Add spiralized zoodles, cherry tomato and season with salt when needed. You might need to cut the zoodles shorter when they are too long. Cook for another 1 minute then turn off the heat.

8. Serve the chicken zoodles with spiced cashews and fresh basil leaves

DAY 7

Breakfast: Keto breakfast pizza (Serves 2/25mins) (page 24)

Calories: 454 kcal

Carbs:26g

Protein:24g

Fat: 35g

INGREDIENTS

- Grated cauliflower (2 cups)
- Coconut flour (2 tbsp)
- Salt (1/2 tsp)
- Salt (1/2 tsp)
- 4 eggs
- Psyllium husk powder (1 tbsp)
- Smoked salmon, herbs, spinach, avocado, and olive oil (as toppings)

HOW TO COOK

1. Preheat oven to 350oF or 170oC. Line a sheet pan or pizza tray with some parchment paper

2. Add all the ingredients (except toppings) into a mixing bowl. Mix until well combined then set aside for about 5 minutes.

3. Carefully power mixture onto a pan then mold into a round and even pizza crust with your hands

4. Bake in the oven for about 15 minutes until it is fully cooked

5. Remove from oven and top with desired toppings. To be served warm.
   Lunch : Low carb mini Mexican meatzas (page 42)

Dinner : 3-Cheese Chicken and Cauliflower Lasagne (page 58)

DAY 8

Breakfast : Keto breakfast burrito (page 25)

Lunch : Spicy kimchi ahi poke (serves 10/4mins) (page 43)

INGREDIENTS

- Ahi tuna (sushi-grade) diced roughly to about 1 inch
- Soy sauce (1 tbsp)
- Sesame oil (1/2 tsp)
- Mayo (1/4 cup)
- Sriracha (2 tbsp)
- Ripe avocado (1, diced)
- Kimchi (1/2 cup)
- Green onion (chopped)
- Sesame seeds

HOW TO COOK

1. Add diced tuna into a medium-sized mixing bowl

2. Add sesame oil, mayo sriracha and soy sauce to this bowl. Toss to mix Ingredients

3. To this bowl, add kimchi and diced avocado then gently mix

4. Serve as topping for salad greens, traditional rice or cauliflower rice. It can be chopped with sesame seeds and green onion.

Dinner : Creamy Tuscan garlic chicken (page 60)

DAY 9

Breakfast : Extra crisp cinnamon toast crunch cereal (page 26)

Lunch : Cinnamon pork chops & mock apples (page 44)

Dinner : Baked chicken with tarragon cream
(Serves 4/30mins) (page 61)

Calories: 151.6kcal

Carbs: 3.4g

Protein 30g

Fat 2g

INGREDIENTS

- 1 tablespoon extra-virgin olive oil
- 4 (about 1.2kg) chicken Marylands
- 15g butter
- 1 large red onion, halved, cut into thin wedges
- 80ml (1/3) dry white wine
- 80ml (1/3) Massel salt reduced chicken style liquid stock
- 300g (2 cups) frozen broad beans
- 80ml (1/3 cup) pouring cream
- 1/3 cup fresh tarragon leaves, plus extra, to serve

HOW TO COOK

1. Preheat oven to 200C/180C fan-forced. Heat half the oil in a large, flameproof, ovenproof roasting pan over medium heat. Season the chicken. Cook, skin side down, for 4-5 minutes or until golden. Turn and cook for a further 2 minutes. Transfer to a plate. Pour off and discard fat from the pan.

2. Heat the butter and remaining oil in the pan over medium-low heat. Cook onion, turning, for 2 minutes or until golden. Add the wine. Simmer for 1 minute. Add stock. Simmer for 1 minute. Remove the heat.

3. Place the chicken on top of the onion. Bake for 30 minutes or until chicken is cooked through. Turn off the oven. Line a baking tray with baking paper. Transfer chicken to prepared tray. Place in the oven to keep warm.

4. Meanwhile, place the broad beans in a heatproof bowl. Cover with boiling water. Stand for 2 minutes. Drain. Refresh under cold running water. Peel.

5. Return to medium heat. Bring it to a simmer. Simmer for 2 minutes or until slightly reduced. Add a cream. Simmer for 2-3 minutes or until slightly reduced. Add the cream. Simmer for 2-3 minutes or until slightly thickened. Add the tarragon. Simmer for 1 minute. Remove chicken to the pan. Sprinkle with remaining broad beans and extra tarragon.

6. Serve with 1 chopped avocado and mixed salad leaves to increase the ratio of fat to protein and carbs.

3-WEEKS WEIGHT LOSS PLAN: HOW TO LOSE UP TO 11 POUNDS IN 21 WEEKS?

93

DAY 10

Breakfast: Oil-free blueberry streusel scones
(serves 12/40mins) (page 28)

Calories:122kcal

Carbs:6g

Protein:5g

Fat:10g

INGREDIENTS

For scones:

- Almond flour (2 cups)
- Baking powder (1 tsp)
- Ground stevia (1/4 tsp)
- Himalayan rock salt (a pinch)
- Fresh blueberries (1 cup)
- 1 egg
- Almond milk (2 tbsp)

For Streusel topping

- Egg white (1 tbsp)
- Silvered almonds (1/4 cup)
- Ground cinnamon (1/2 tsp)
- Stevia (a pinch)

HOW TO COOK

1. Preheat oven to about 375oF or 180oC. Line baking sheet with parchment paper

2. Mix all the ingredients for the streusel topping in a small bowl

3. Mix almond flour, salt baking powder, and stevia in a large bowl then mix thoroughly

4. Add in blueberries until well coated with the flour mixture. Set this aside

5. Mix egg and almond milk in a bowl, add the wet mixture to your flour mixture, continue to stir until fully mixed and the dough can be kneaded with no problems

6. Shape dough to form 12 small cones about 1/2 inch each then place on prepared sheet. Press the topping on top of each scone

7. Bake for about 20 to 22 minutes or until color turns golden

8. Leave to cool for about 10 minutes then serve.

Lunch: Caprese Eggplant Panini with Lemon Basil Aioli (page 45)

Dinner: 20-minute Low Carb Turkey and Pepper (page 62)

DAY 11

Breakfast: Keto chocolate muffins (page 29)

Lunch: Slow cooking keto chili (serves 6/8hrs 15mins) (page 46)

Calories:387kcal

Carbs: 7.2g

Protein:33g

Fat: 24g

INGREDIENTS

- ground beef (1 lb/0.45kg)
- Ground sausage (1 lb/0.45kg)
- Chopped Green bell pepper (1, medium)
- Diced tomato (1 can, 14.5oz)
- Tomato paste (1 can, 6oz)
- Chilli powder (1 tbsp)
- Ground cumin (1/2 tbsp)
- Garlic cloves (3 to 4) minced
- Water (1/3 cup)

HOW TO COOK

1. Brown ground beef and sausage
2. Drain. Keep half of the fat for later
3. Place cooked sausage and ground beef in a crockpot
4. Add the fat dripping and all other ingredients then mix well.
5. Cover the crockpot with the lid and cook for 6 to 8 hours
6. Remove and serve topped with cheese, sour cream and green onions

Dinner: Broccoli rice with chicken coconut curry (page 64)

DAY 12

Breakfast : Buttery coconut flour waffles (page 30)

Lunch : Keto broccoli soup with turmeric and ginger (page 47)

Dinner: Smoked salmon egg pots (Serves 4/20mins) (page 97)

Calories: 285kcal

Carbs: 1.4g

Protein 27.8g

Fat 18.9g

INGREDIENTS

- ◆ 250g smoked salmon slices
- ◆ 6 large eggs, beaten
- ◆ 1 tablespoon chives, chopped
- ◆ 3 tablespoon crème Fraiche

- ◆ Salt and black pepper
- ◆ 1 tablespoon horseradish sauce
- ◆ Lemon juice
- ◆ Salad leaves to serve

HOW TO COOK

1. Preheat the oven to 180C/160C fan-forced. Grease four ramekins with a little oil, use the smoked salmon to line the inside of each ramekin leaving no gaps and leaving enough hanging over the edges to cover the tops later.

2. Cut any remaining salmon into small pieces after lining and add the beaten egg along with the chives. Season with salt and black pepper.

3. Pour the egg mixture into the lined ramekins and gently fold over the salmon.

4. Place the ramekins on a baking tray, pour water in the tray to around 5cm depth, then bake in the oven for 15-20 minutes or until set and firm to touch.

5. Mix the black pepper, lemon juice, horseradish, and crème Fraiche.

6. Remove the water once the eggs are cooked and turn upside down on a plate. Remove the ramekin and serve with salad leaves and hollandaise.

DAY 13

Breakfast: Keto breakfast tacos with bacon and guacamole (serves 2/15mins) (page 98)

Calories:387kcal

Carbs: 9g

Protein: 11g

Fat: 35g

INGREDIENTS

- Brain octane oil (1 tablespoon)
- Pastured raised eggs (2)
- Grass-fed ghee (1 tbsp)
- Organic avocado (1, medium)
- Himalayan salt (1/2 tsp)
- Organic romaine lettuce-chopped (1/4 cup)
- Cooked pastured bacon (2 slices)
- Organic sweet potatoes-diced and cooked (3 tbsp)
- Organic micro cilantro (optional for garnish)

HOW TO COOK

1. Heat small skillet on medium heat then add 1 tbsp of ghee
2. Into the skillet, crack one egg then pierce the yolk
3. Cook for about 1 to 2 minutes on each side until solid
4. Remove egg from pan and place on a parchment paper-lined plate
5. Repeat this for all the eggs
6. Mash avocado along with Brain Octane oil and Himalayan pink salt in a small bowl. Divide this mixture evenly then spread on each egg taco shell
7. Top each with the romaine lettuce
8. On each taco, place a slice of bacon and half of diced potatoes. You can also garnish with cilantro and add a tiny sprinkle of Himalayan salt
9. Fold in half to form a taco.

Lunch: Easy keto asiago cauliflower rice (page 48)

Dinner: Beef and broccoli bowls with sunshine sauce (page 66)

DAY 14

Breakfast: Bacon & egg fat bombs (page 32)

Lunch: Low carb chicken Philly cheesesteak bowl (serves 3/25mins) (page 49)

Calories: 263 kcal

Carbs: 5g

Protein:27g

Fat: 13g

INGREDIENTS

- Chicken breasts (10 oz/1.2kg)- boneless
- Worcestershire sauce (2 tbsp)
- Onion powder (1/2 tsp)
- Garlic powder (1/2 tsp)
- Dash ground pepper
- Olive oil (2 tsp)

- Fresh or frozen onion (1/2 cup)
- Minced garlic (1/2 tsp)
- Provolone cheese (3 slices)
- Diced bell pepper (1/2 cup)
- 10 oz boneless chicken breasts (about 2)

HOW TO COOK

1. Cut chicken breasts into thin slices and place in a bowl.

2. Add Worcestershire sauce, ground pepper, onion powder, and garlic powder then stir until chicken is fully coated

3. Heat 1 tsp oil in an oven-proof skillet. To this add the chicken pieces and cook for about 5 minutes until well browned. Turn pieces over, cook for 2 to 3 more minutes until browned before removing from skillet

4. Add the rest of the olive oil to a warm skillet, add onions, garlic and bell pepper. Cook while stirring continuously until tender (for about 3 minutes)

5. Turn down the heat and return chicken to the skillet, add veggies and stir to combine. Add in the sliced cheese and cover skillet for about 3 minutes until cheese melts

Dinner: Bacon avocado salad (page 68)

DAY 15

Breakfast: Bacon and egg breakfast muffins (page 35)

Lunch: Easy keto egg salad (page 50)

Dinner: Ground beef and cabbage stir fry
(serves 2/25mins) (page 69)

Calories: 301kcal

Carbs: 8.3g

Protein 32.7g

Fat 15.2g

INGREDIENTS

- 1 pound extra-lean ground beef
- 9-ounce bag coleslaw mix, purple cabbage, carrot, and shredded cabbage.
- Sesame oil (1tbsp)
- Rice vinegar (2 tablespoons)
- Garlic, minced (2 cloves)
- ¼ tbsp red pepper flakes
- Soy sauce ¼ cup (to replace soy, use coconut aminos, tamari, or wheat)
- ½ tablespoon salt
- Scallions for garnish (Chopped, optional)
- Grated fresh ginger (1tbsp)
- ¼ tablespoon ground black pepper

HOW TO COOK

1. In a small bowl, combine the rice vinegar, soy sauce, black pepper, red pepper falkes, and salt.
2. Prepare a large skillet and heat the sesame oil over high-medium heat. Include the beef and let it cook for about b9 mins till it is browned.
3. Add ginger and garlic and cook for about 2mins.
4. Mix the soy sauce and coleslaw mix into the skiller. Let it cook for about 7mins. Stir to soften the cabbage.
5. Use chopped scallions as garnish.

DAY 16

Breakfast: Bulletproof coffee egg latte (serves 1/12mins) (page 18)

Calories: 331Kcal

Carbs: 4.5g

Protein: 24g

Fat: 25g

INGREDIENTS:

- Black coffee (8 oz/227g)
- Grass-fed butter or ghee (1 to 2 tbsp)
- Brain octane oil (1 to 2 tbsp)
- Pastured raised egg-2 eggs
- Vanilla collagen protein (1 scoop)
- Ceylon Cinnamon (1/4 teaspoon)

HOW TO COOK

6. Blend eggs, oil, butter, and mix with cinnamon
7. Add coffee then blend for 45 seconds more on high speed
8. Include collagen protein then blend for 5 more seconds at low speed
9. Add cinnamon for topping

Lunch: Easy shrimp avocado salad with tomatoes and feta (page 38)

Dinner: Baked chicken with tarragon cream (page 61)

DAY 17

Breakfast: Coconut flour crepes (page 20)

Lunch: Chicken enchilada (serves 4/50mins) (page 39)

Calories: 568kcal

Carbs: 6g

Protein: 38g

Fat: 40g

INGREDIENTS

- 2 tablespoons Coconut oil
- 1 lbs/0.45kg Boneless and skinless chicken thigh
- ¾ cup Red enchilada sauce

For Toppings:
- 1 whole diced avocado
- 1 cup Shredded cheese
- 1 chopped Roma tomato

- ¼ cup water Water
- (1 can, 4 oz/500g) Diced green chilies

- ½ cup Sour cream
- ¼ cup Chopped pickled jalapenos

HOW TO COOK

1. Set a pot and melt the coconut oil over medium heat or in a dutch oven. Sear chickeni until it is lightly brown in oil.

2. Add water and enchilada sauce. Add green chiles and onion and reduce the heat. Cover it up and let it simmer for about 25mins until chicken is well cooked.

3. Remove chicken carefully and place on a flat surface, chop or shred chicken and transfer it back to the pot. Uncover the pot and let it simmer for 10mins.

4. Set it down from the oven and serve with jalapeno, avocado, sour cream, tomato, and chees for topping. It can be served with cauliflower rice as well.

   Dinner: Ground beef and cabbage stir fry (page 69)

DAY 18

Breakfast: Extra crisp cinnamon toast crunch cereal (page 26)

Lunch: Easy keto lasagna stuffed portobellos (page 40)

Dinner: Sunshine sauce with broccoli bowl
and beef (serves 4/20mins) (page 66)

Calories: 388kcal

Carbs: 9.3g

Protein 30g

Fat 29g

INGREDIENTS

Broccoli

- Fine salt (1/2 tbsp)
- Avocado oil (1 tbsp)
- Cut 4 broccoli crowns into florets

Beef

- Cooking fat (1 tbsp)
- Granulated garlic (1tbsp)
- Fine salt (1 tbsp)
- Coconut aminos (1 tbsp)
- Ground beef lean grass fed (1 pound 85%)

Sunshine sauce

- Bone broth (1/4 cup)
- Ground ginger (1 tbsp)
- Ground pepper (1 tsp)
- Sunflower seed butter oil (2 tbsp)
- Cooking fat (1 tbsp)
- Coconut aminos (2 tbsp)
- Lemon juice
- 1 Mined green onion
- Fine salt (1/2)
- **Assembling**
- Baby spinach (4 cups) though optional

HOW TO COOK

1. Set oven at 400 °F. Prepare a sheet pan and mix the salt and fat with the broccoli. Spread the fat by massaging it into the florets and spread them on the sheet to prevent overcrowding.

2. While the oven pre-heats, put in the sheet pan and set the timer at 20mins.

3. Over medium heat, heat a skillet and add the fat when the temperature is reached.

4. Add garlic and salt to the skiller and crumble gound beef in it. Stir continuously and whisk till it is crumbly or browned. Increase the heat and put coconut aminos.

5. Cook and stir continuously till crispy or dark brown.

6. In the meanwhile, set a small saucepot over medium heat.

7. Melt the fat than the sunflower seed, stirring until smooth.

8. Addd the ground ginger, salt aminos, and bone broth. Stir continuously till it mixes well.

9. Set down from the heat and add lemon juice. Stir till it is smooth.

10. Mix in the green onions. Set aside.

11. In a bowl, make a bed of 4 large baby spinach. In the bowl, add the ground beef and broccoli florets. To complete the assembling, spoon the sauce over it.

Breakfast: Keto breakfast pizza (serves 2/25mins) (page 24)

Calories: 454 kcal

Carbs:26g

Protein:24g

Fat: 35g

INGREDIENTS

- 2 cups Gratedcauliflower
- ½ tablespoon Salt
- 2 tablespoons Coconut flour
- 4 eggs
- ½ tablespoon Salt

- 1 tablespoon Psyllium husk powder
- Smoked salmon, herbs, spinach, olive oil as topping and avocado

HOW TO COOK

1. Preheat oven to 350oF or 170oC. Line a sheet pan or pizza tray with some parchment paper

2. Add all the ingredients in a mixing bowl apart from the toppings. Mix until it is combined and leave it for 5 minutes.

3. Carefully power mixture onto a pan then mould into a round and even pizza crust with your hands

4. Bake in the oven for about 15 minutes and leave until it is fully cooked.

5. Take it out of the open and use it with any topping of your choice. Enjoy warm.

Lunch: Low carb mini mexican meatzas (page 42)

Dinner: Broccoli rice with Chicken Coconut Curry (page 64)

DAY 20

Breakfast: Buttery coconut flour waffles (page 30)

Lunch: Easy keto asiago cauliflower rice (serves 4/15mins) (page 48)

Calories: 250kcal

Carbs: 5.6g

Protein:7.1g

Fat: 21.7g

INGREDIENTS

- ◆ Riced cauliflower (3 cups)
- ◆ Shredded Asiago cheese (1 cup)
- ◆ Heavy cream (3/4 cup)
- ◆ Fresh basil (chopped, optional)

HOW TO COOK

1. Add riced cauliflower into a saute pan. Add 2 tbsp of water, cover then cook for about 5 minutes

2. Add cheese and cream and mix until cheese melts

3. Taste to see if cauliflower is ready

4. Remove from heat and serve. You can add freshly chopped basil to top
    Dinner: Baked chicken with tarragon cream (page 61)

DAY 21

Breakfast: Keto chocolate cake donuts (page 88)

Lunch: Chicken tomato zoodles with spiced cashew (page 57)

Dinner: Garlic chicken creamy Tuscan (serves 4-6/30mins) (page 60)

Calories: 487.7kcal

Carbs: 7.3g

Protein 33.8g

Fat 35.8g

INGREDIENTS

- 1 ½ pounds boneless skinless chicken breasts, thinly sliced
- 2 tablespoons olive oil
- 1 cup heavy cream
- ½ cup chicken broth

- 1 teaspoon garlic powder
- Parmesan cheese (1/2 cup)
- Chopped spinach (1 cup)
- Sun-dried tomatoes (½ cup)
- 1 tablespoon Italian seasoning

HOW TO COOK

1. Add sufficient amount of olive oil to a large skillet. On high-medium heat, cook the chicken for about 5mins till it browns on each side or you till the pink center is no longer visible.

2. Prepare a separate plate and set the chicken aside after removing it from the skillet.

3. Add the chicken broth, garlic powder, heavy cream, parmesan cheese, and Italian seasoning. To make it thicken, whisk it over medium-high heat.

4. Add sundried tomatoes and spinach, let it simmer to make the spinach wilt.

5. Return the chicken to the pan and add pastea to serving if you want.

The opinions and ideas of the author contained in this publication are designed to educate the reader in an informative and helpful manner. While we accept that the instructions will not suit every reader, it is only to be expected that the recipes might not gel with everyone. Use the book responsibly and at your own risk. This work with all its contents, does not guarantee correctness, completion, quality or correctness of the provided information. Always check with your medical practitioner should you be unsure whether to follow a low carb eating plan. Misinformation or misprints cannot be completely eliminated. Human error is real!

Cover: oliviaprodesign

Cover Photo: zarzamora / shutterstock.com

DISCLAIMER

KT-382-830

WITHDRAWN

Stories

Tiny Pig

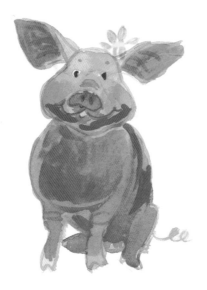

by Iris Josiah

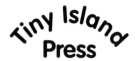

Published in the United Kingdom by:

Tiny Island Press
1 Bromley Lane
Chislehurst
Kent BR7 6LH, U.K

Copyright © Iris Josiah, 2012
Illustrations by Jane-Ann Cameron
Design & layout by Re-shape Invent

All rights reserved. No portion of this book may be reproduced, stored in a retrieval system or transmitted at anytime, in any form or by any means mechanical, electronic, photocopying, recording or otherwise without the prior, written permission of the copyright holder.

The right of Iris Josiah to be identified as the author of this work has been asserted by her in accordance with the Copyright, Designs and Patents Act 1988, sections 77 and 78.

A CIP record of this book is available from the British Library
Printed 1 November 2012

ISBN: 978-0-9572728-1-1
Printed in the United Kingdom

WESTERN ISLES LIBRARIES	
34134000847365	
Bertrams	20/12/2012
	£8.99

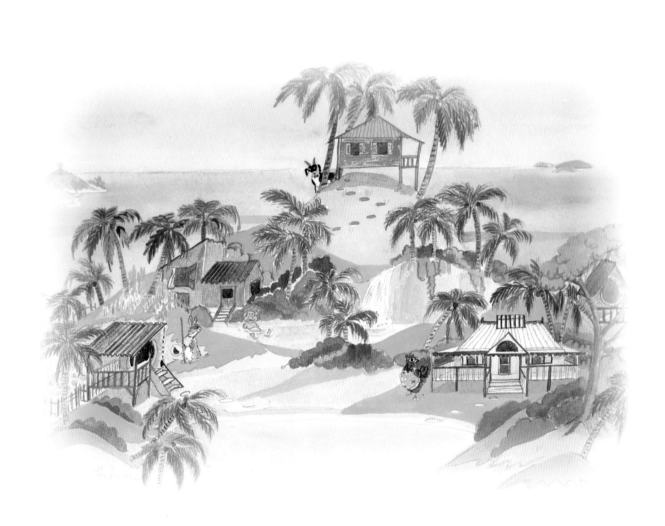

Tiny Pig was a playful little pig
that lived on Tiny Island.

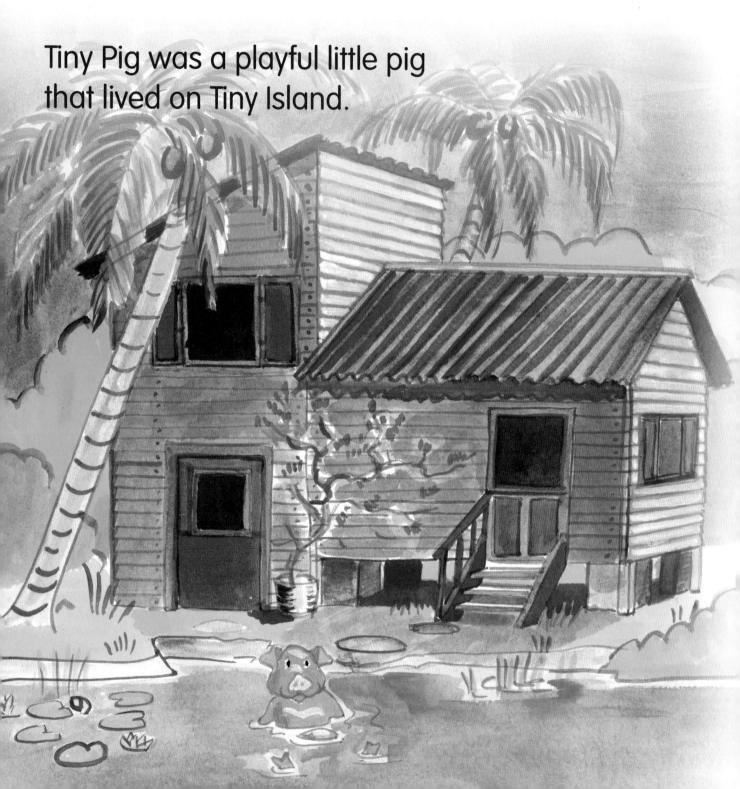

Tiny Pig loved to play and would lie in the mud for a very long time ROLLING and ROLLING, OVER and OVER and OVER.

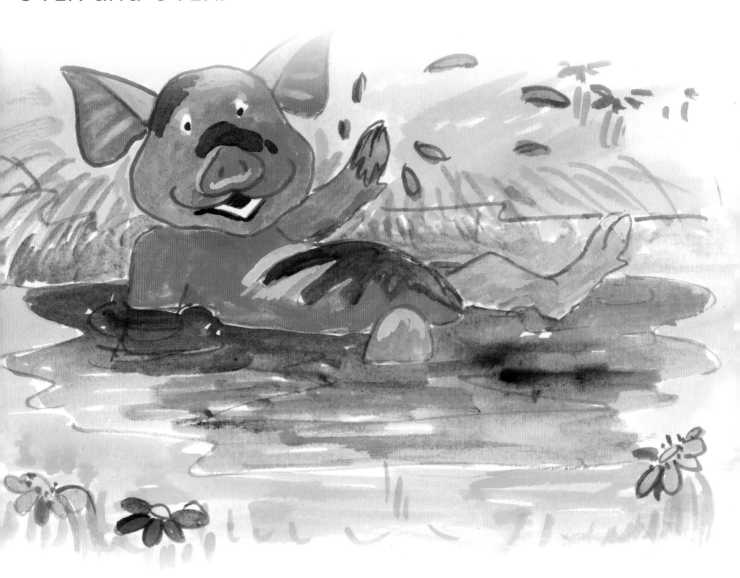

But Tiny Pig had not played in the mud for many days. Instead, he had become a very worried little pig.

He WORRIED and WORRIED and WORRIED because of a rumour in his village.

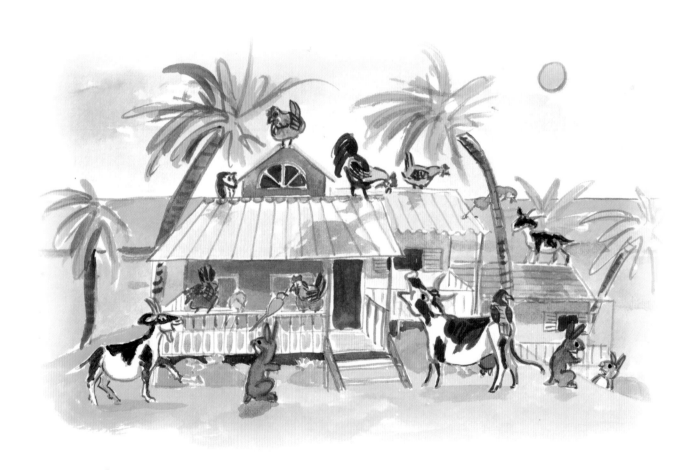

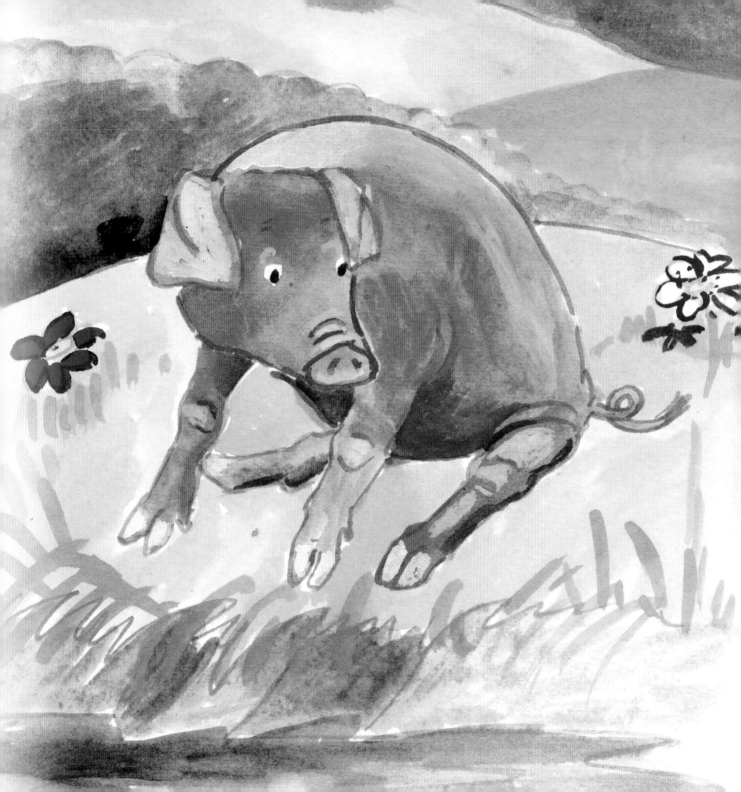

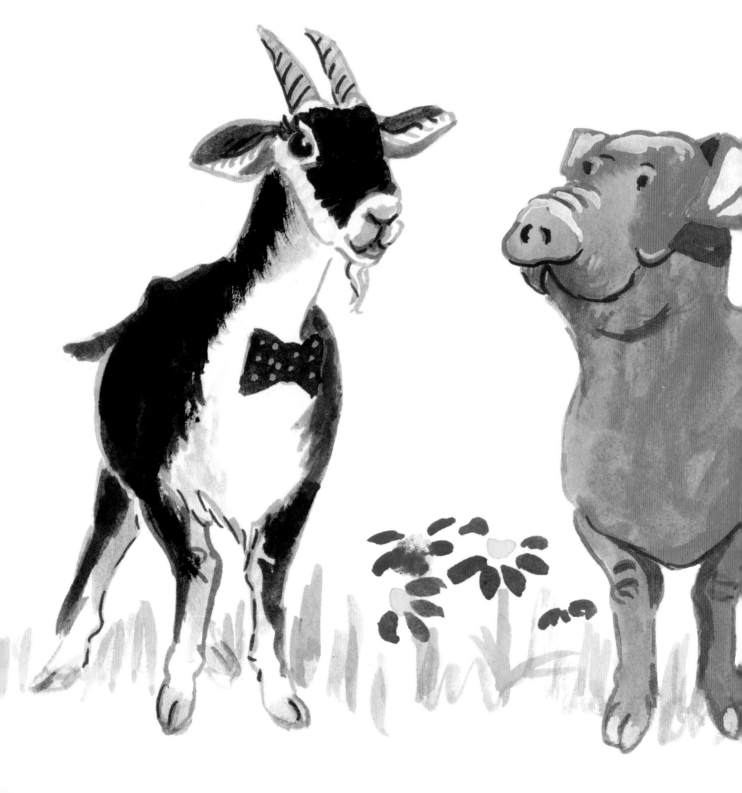

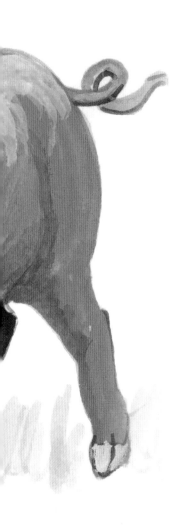

'There is a rumour in the village that the Great Wise Village Pig is your father,' his little friend Tiny Goat said to him.

'No, this could not be,' replied Tiny Pig in amazement as he tried desperately to appear untroubled.

But he was very troubled. So troubled was Tiny Pig that he WORRIED and WORRIED and WORRIED and had not slept comfortably since speaking to Tiny Goat.

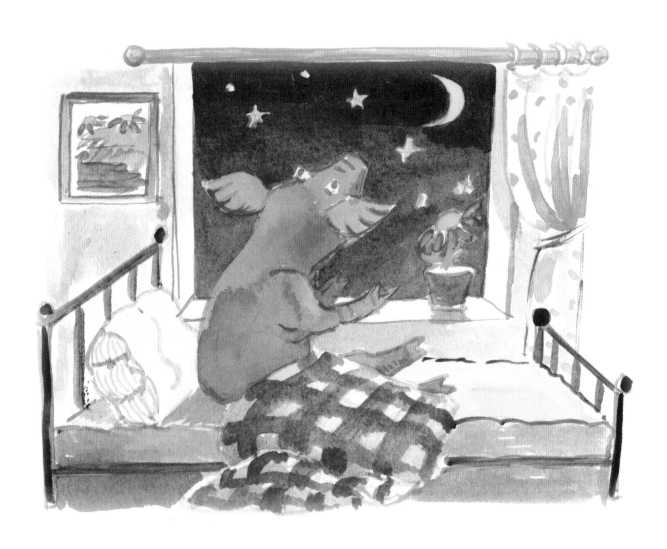

'I shall have a rest,' he mumbled to himself as he STRETCHED and STRETCHED and STRETCHED.

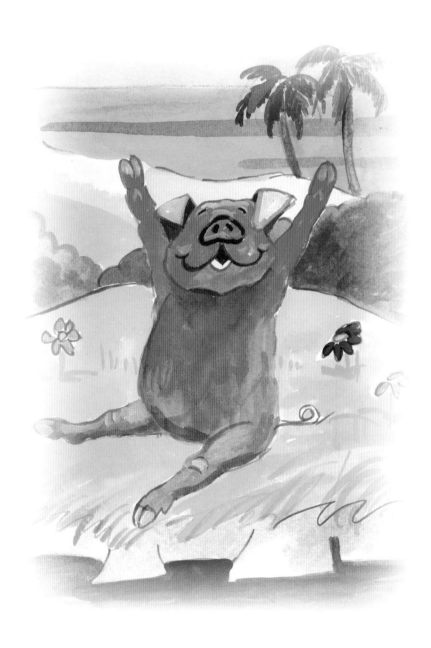

And he felt fast asleep.

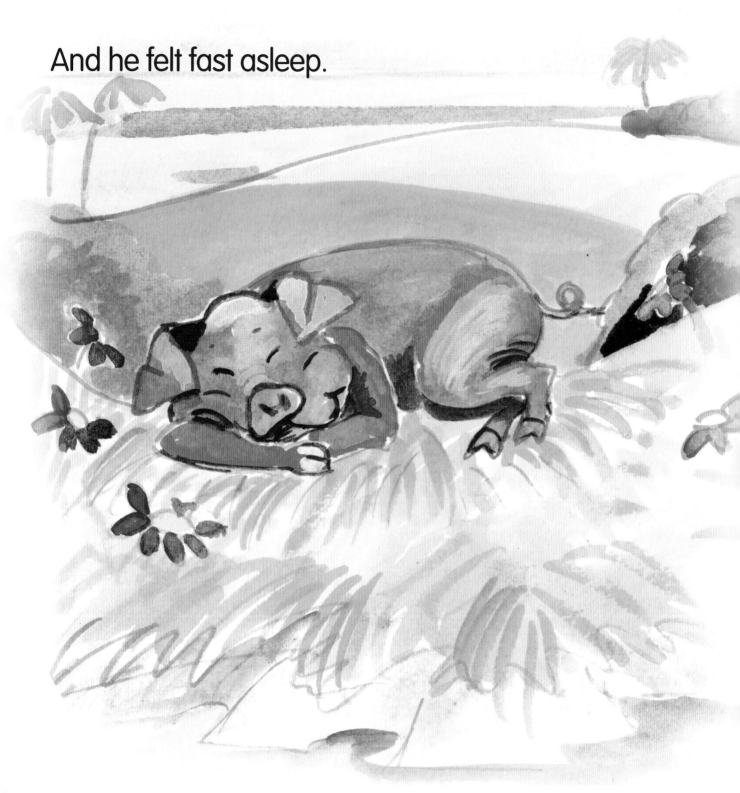

Soon, he was wide awake. And to his surprise,
he began to play in the mud. OVER and OVER he rolled.
And he was not worried anymore.

'I must go to see the Great Wise Village Pig,'
he smiled to himself.

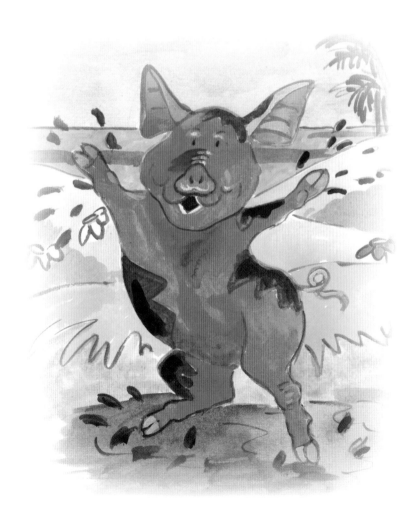

Without a word to anyone, he made his way through his front gate and hurried off to find the Great Wise Village Pig.

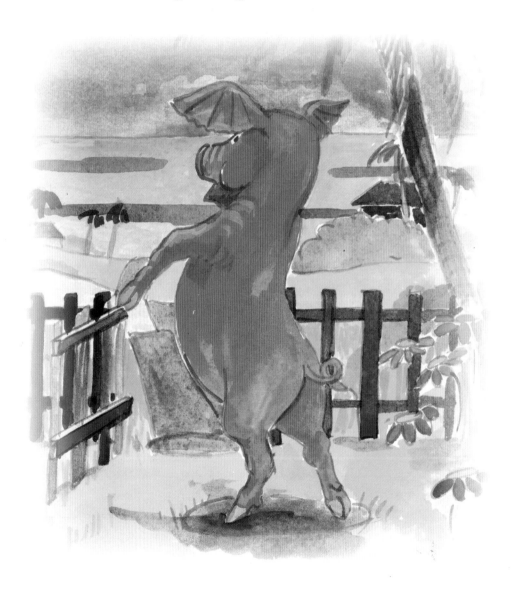

He met Tiny Hen and many of his friends.
'Good-day,' he said and on he went.

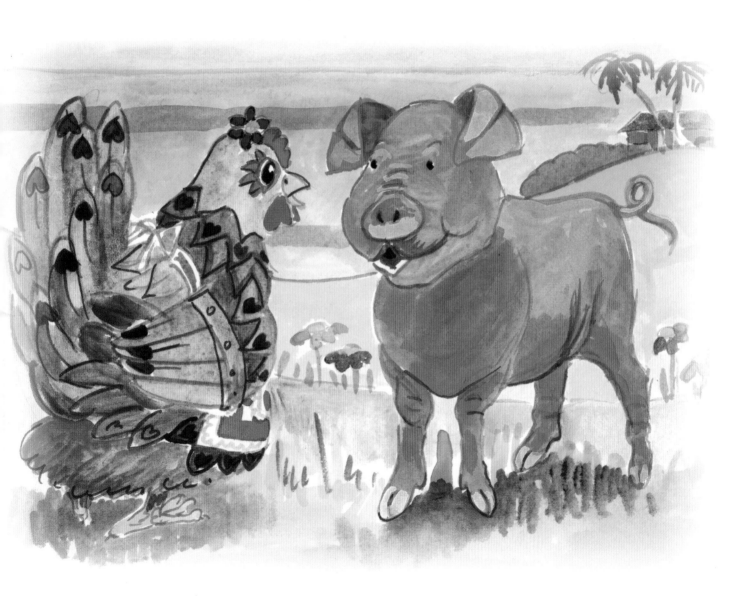

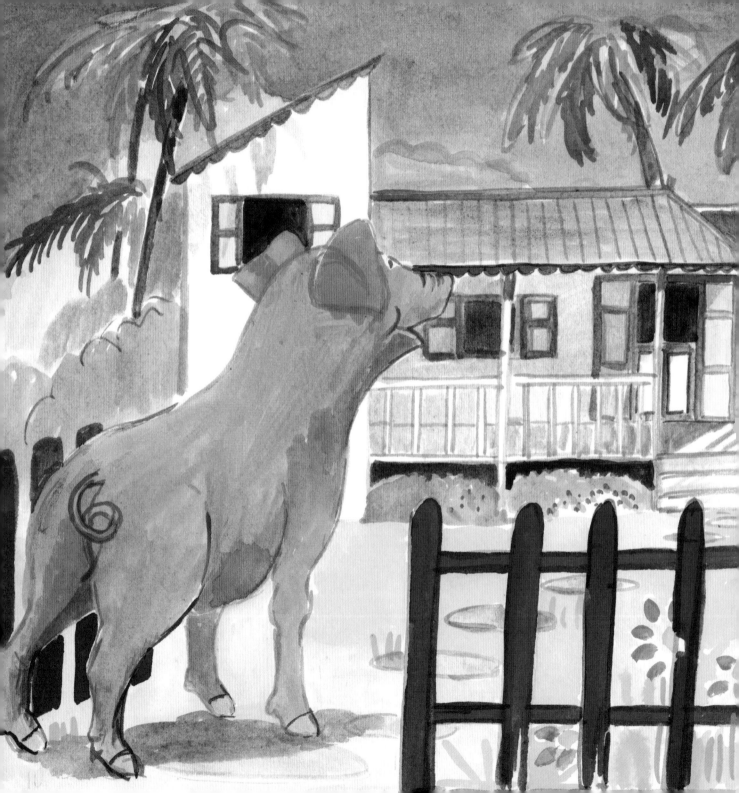

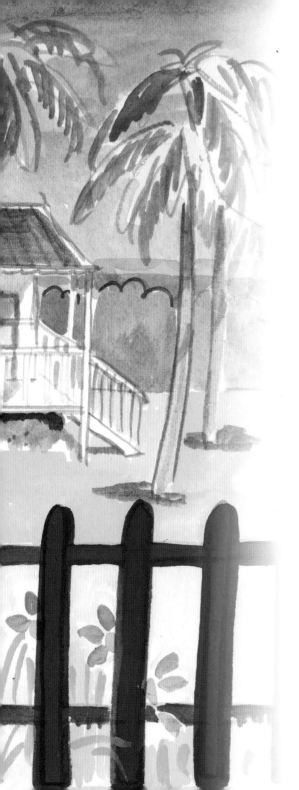

Then he came to the Great Wise Village Pig's house. It was the most beautiful house in the village and the most beautiful one he had ever seen.

He pushed the gates open, entered the yard and made his way to the back. And there to meet him was the Great Wise Village Pig.

'Good-day,' said Tiny Pig.

'Good-day,' replied the Great Wise Village Pig.

'There is something I must ask you,' went on Tiny Pig. 'There is a rumour in the village that you are my father. Tell me, is this true?'

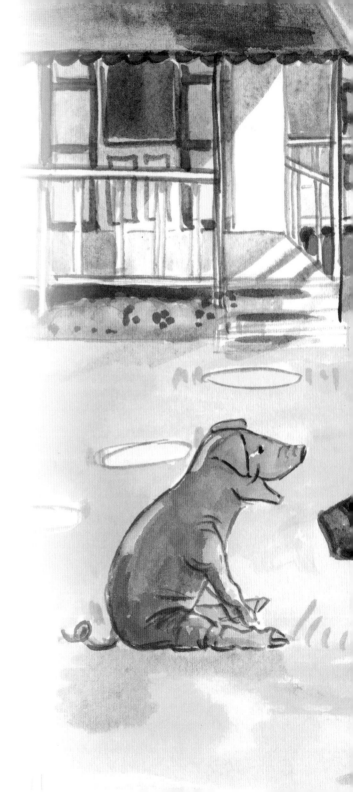

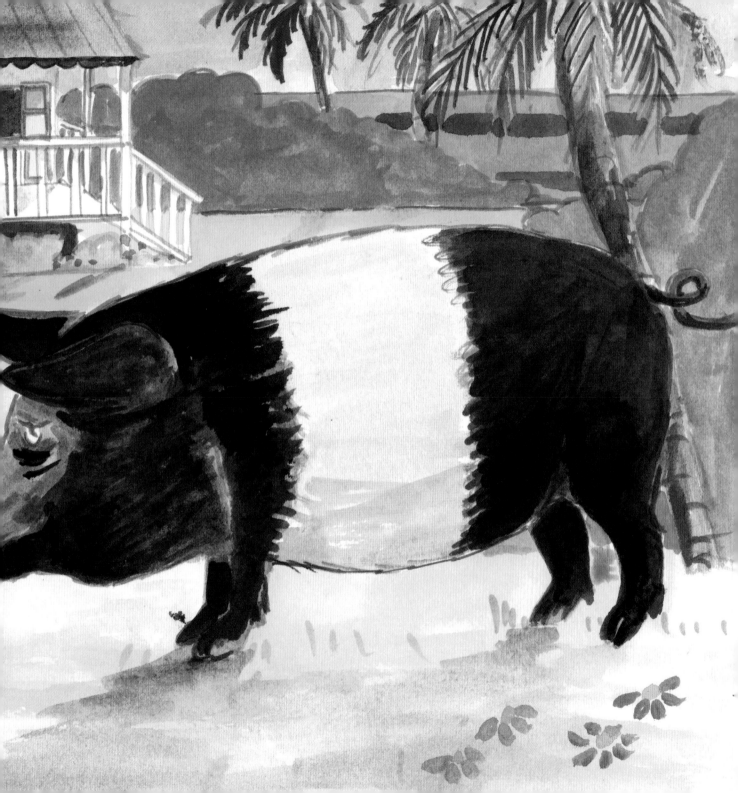

And the Great Wise Village Pig whispered softly, 'Yes.'

'Oh father,' cried Tiny Pig.

And he CRIED and CRIED and CRIED. And he hugged and kissed the Great Wise Village Pig. And they TALKED and TALKED and TALKED.

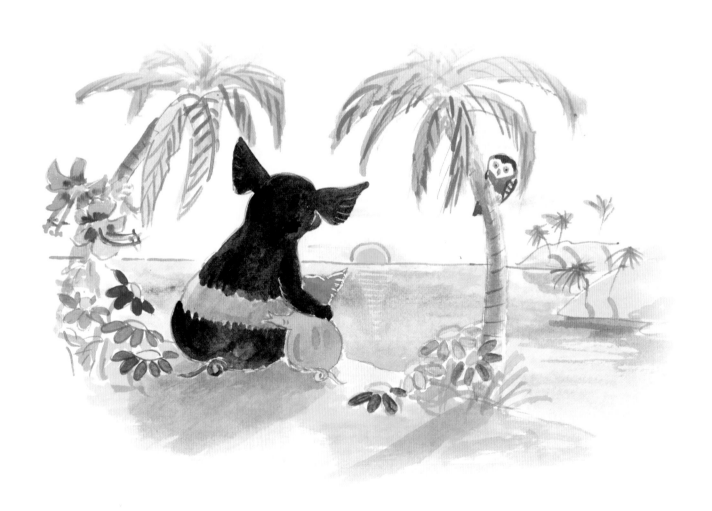

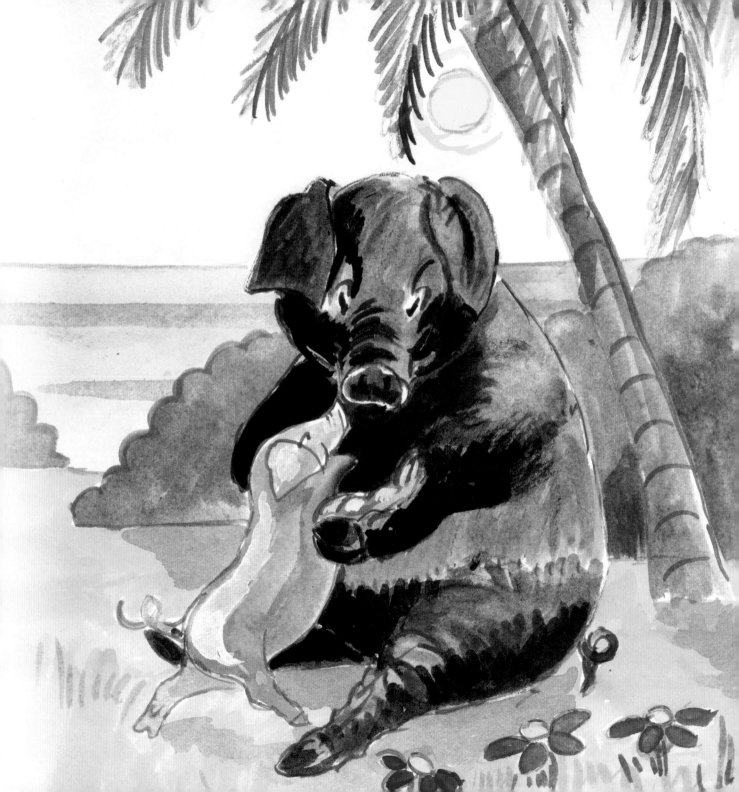

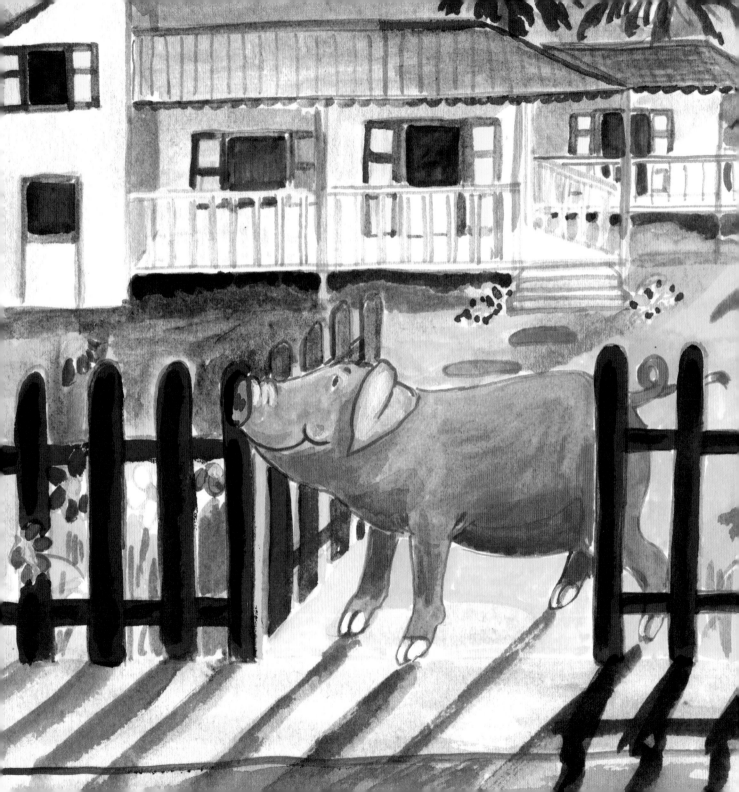

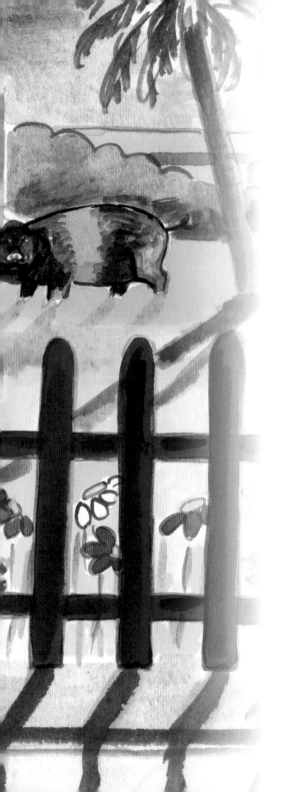

Soon, it was dusk and Tiny Pig bade the Great Wise Pig goodbye.

'You must come and see me again,' said the Great Wise Pig.

'Yes, I shall,' said Tiny Pig.

And he made his way to the front yard, through the gates and onto the sidewalk. He stopped for a while and bowed his head.

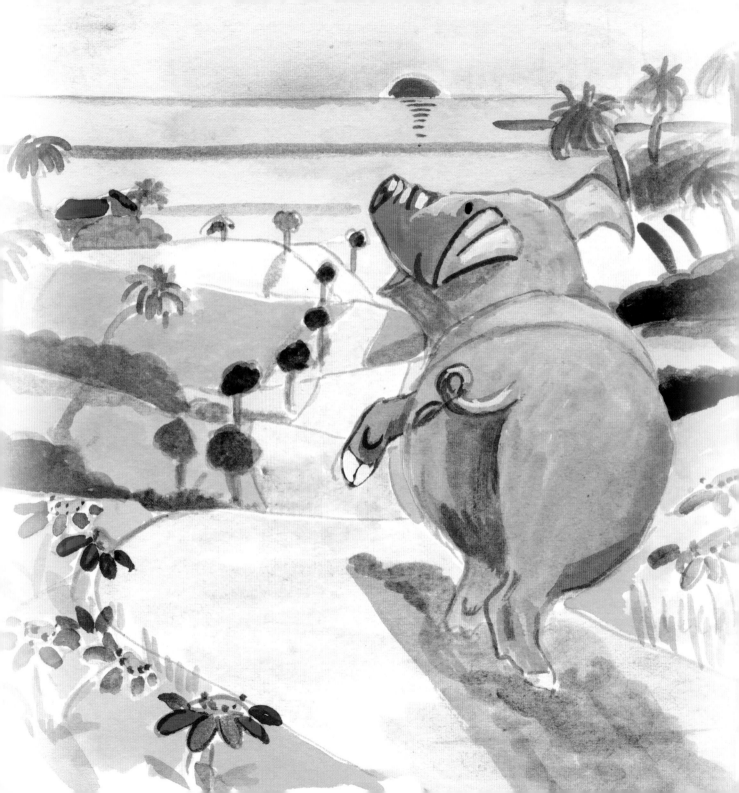

'Oink, oink,' grunted Tiny Pig playfully. And off he went.

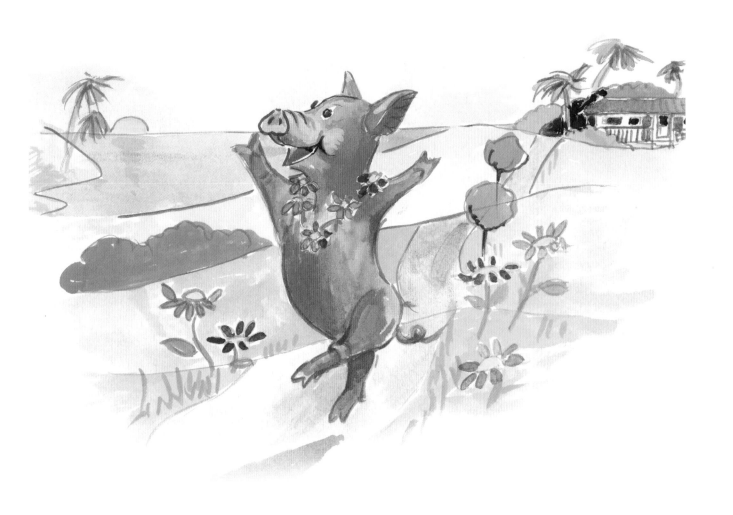

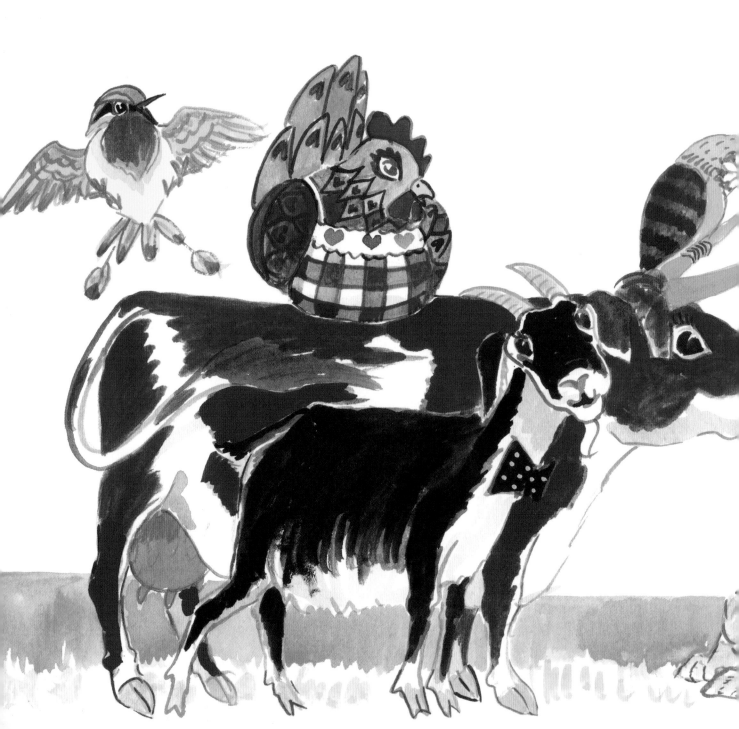

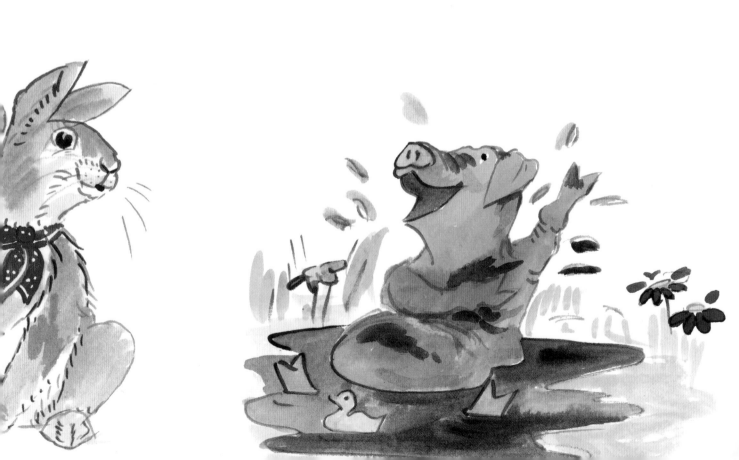

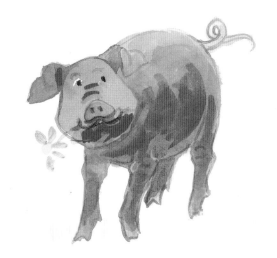